The Child with Cancer
– Nursing Care

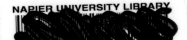

The Child with Cancer – Nursing Care

Edited by
Jenny Thompson
SRN RSCN OncNursCert FETC
Paediatric Services Manager
The Royal Marsden Hospital, Sutton, Surrey

With ten contributors

Scutari Press
London

A division of Scutari Projects, the publishing
company of the Royal College of Nursing

First published 1990

British Library Cataloguing in Publication Data

The child with cancer – nursing care.
　1. Cancer patients.　Children.　Nursing
　I. Thompson, Jenny
　610.7362

　　ISBN 1-871364-36-1

Typeset by Litho Link Limited, Welshpool, Powys, Wales
Printed and bound in Great Britain by Henry Ling Limited, Dorchester

Contents

Contributors

Alison Arnfield RSCN RGN OncNursCert HECert FETC
Clinical Nurse Manager, The Hospitals for Sick Children, Great Ormond Street, London

Elspeth L Brewis RSCN SRN SCM
Nursing Officer – Medical, The Royal Hospital for Sick Children, Yorkhill, Glasgow

Steven J Campbell BNurs RHV RSCN NDNCert
Staff Nurse, Professorial Paediatric Ward, Royal Victoria Infirmary, Newcastle upon Tyne; Postgraduate Nursing Research Student, School of Health & Behavioural Science, Newcastle upon Tyne Polytechnic

Anne M Casey RGN RSCN DipN DipNEd
Nurse Teacher – Paediatric Oncology, The Hospitals for Sick Children, Great Ormond Street, London

Margaret Evans RSCN RGN FETC DipN(Lond)
Nurse Specialist – Paediatric Oncology, Southampton General Hospital

Lesley J Geen SRN RSCN
Formerly Ward Sister – Paediatrics, Kingston General Hospital

Jane F A Mashru SRN RSCN
Sister, Princess Chula Ward, The Royal Marsden Hospital, Sutton, Surrey

Anne Nicholson MSc SRN RSCN HVCert RNT
Director of Nursing, The Royal Victoria Infirmary, Newcastle upon Tyne

Nina Patel RGN RHV FWT OncNursCert
Community Liaison/Home Care Sister, The Royal Marsden Hospital, Sutton, Surrey

Beth Sepion RSCN RGN SCM OncNursCert FETC
Senior Nurse Paediatrics, The Royal Marsden Hospital, Sutton, Surrey

Jenny Thompson RGN RSCN OncNursCert FETC
Director of Nursing Services, The Royal Marsden Hospital, London

Preface

Childhood cancer has assumed a greater significance in modern paediatric practice because the control of other causes of death in childhood, notably infection and perinatal problems, has meant that childhood cancer is the most important fatal disease in children after the first year of life.

Childhood cancers differ from adult cancers. The common adult cancers such as those of the lung, breast and cervix rarely occur in children, but bone marrow, germ cell tumours and Wilms' tumour (nephroblastoma) occur almost exclusively in children. With the development of specialist centres, rapid advances in the treatment of childhood cancer have occurred, and the stage has now been reached where between 60 and 70 per cent of all children diagnosed as having cancer can be cured.

Childhood cancer must be viewed as a family illness; support for the child and his family is of paramount importance. Along with advances in treatment, concern for the psychosocial impact and the quality of life assumes particular importance as the prospects for survival increase: thus, the focus of this book is the physical and psychosocial care of children and their families through all phases of treatment.

The psychological, social and other non-medical needs of sick children and their families have not been forgotten in the preoccupation with highly technical treatments and hospital routines. It is recognised throughout the book that meeting these needs is just as important for the health of the children and their families.

The contributors to *The Child with Cancer – Nursing Care* are all nurses whose collective experience extends over the whole range of paediatric oncology, and the aim of the book is to bring together information on current approaches to the management of childhood cancer. For this reason, basic paediatric care is not included in detail as it is already covered in standard textbooks of paediatric nursing.

Jenny Thompson
1989

Acknowledgements

The editor is grateful for the support of all who made possible the publication of this book. In particular, the support of Dr Alan Craft, Consultant Paediatrician, The Children's Department, The Royal Infirmary, Newcastle upon Tyne, Mr Robert Tiffany, Director of In-Patient Services/Chief Nursing Officer and Mr Phylip Pritchard, former Assistant to the Director of In-Patient Services, at The Royal Marsden Hospital, for their continuing encouragement and assistance, is acknowledged.

Appreciation is due to Mrs Miranda Morgan for her initial secretarial support and to Mrs Lela Novak who has prepared so many drafts and revisions.

Special thanks are extended to staff in the Photographic Department at The Royal Marsden Hospital, who so promptly responded to requests for photographic material.

To the parents and children I extend my gratitude for their permission to reproduce photographs, poems and an illustration.

To Mr Graham Dean for his support and understanding of the time devoted to the preparation of this book.

JT

1
Childhood Cancer – An Overview

Patterns of illness in children have changed dramatically over the past few decades with many of the infectious diseases being virtually eliminated (Table 1.1). Other illnesses have emerged to take their place and there has been a consequent change in the organisation of care for sick children in hospital. There has been a move away from all paediatric units treating the full spectrum of illnesses to one of much greater centralisation and specialisation, particularly for rare conditions. This is well exemplified by the changes that have taken place in the care of children with malignant disease. Childhood cancer has become the most important fatal disease in children after the first year of life and is a major reason for admission to hospital. The most common causes of death in England and Wales in 1985 are shown in Table 1.2.

INCIDENCE

Cancer affects 1 in 600 children before their fifteenth birthday; on a population basis this gives an annual occurrence of 20 per million total population. There are many different types of cancer, approximately one third being leukaemia, one fifth brain tumours and the remainder cancers of various organs, particularly kidney and adrenal, or of specific tissues, e.g. bone or muscle. The most common cancers in children and their incidence are shown in Table 1.3. As can be seen, they are not the same as the common malignant diseases of adults and their treatment and outcome are also very different. A prerequisite for planning and the organisation of services for children with cancer is an accurate knowledge of the prevalence in any particular community. That is why many regions in the United Kingdom have now established children's malignant disease registries. The first of these was established in Manchester in 1954 and this was followed by Newcastle in 1968. In recent years many other regions have opened their own register. A registry not only

1

Table 1.1 Deaths of children aged 1–14 years from various causes (Adapted from Court, 1976. Reproduced by kind permission of HMSO)

Cause	1911–15 No.	1911–15 Rate/million	1931–35 No.	1931–35 Rate/million	1956–60 No.	1956–60 Rate/million	1970–74 No.	1970–74 Rate/million	1976–80 No.	1976–80 Rate/million
Diphtheria	23,380	447	13,820	311	15	0	1	0	0	0
Measles	48,986	936	10,874	254	210	4	111	2	83	1.6
Whooping cough	20,182	385	6,071	137	72	1	7	0	10	0.2
Gastroenteritis	25,560	488	3,485	78	447	9	487	9	137	2.7
Tuberculosis	46,459	887	14,544	327	306	6	71	1	35	0.7
Scarlet fever	9,901	189	2,589	58	7	0	0	0	–	–
Rheumatic fever[a]	3,495	67	2,465	55	139	3	6	0	35	0.7
Cancer	2,388	46	2,853	64	3,971	83	3,743	69	2,931	57.3
Pneumonia and bronchitis	76,643	1,464	28,226	635	3,347	70	2,330	43	1,454	28.4
Accidents	18,500	353	12,126	273	6,736	140	7,214	133	5,273	103.0

[a]The figures are not strictly comparable because of revision of the ICD (International Classification of Disease) Code.

Table 1.2 Major causes of death in childhood: England and Wales 1985

Age-group	0–1		1–4		5–9		10–14		0–14	
	No.	%	No.	%	No.	%	No.	%	No.	%
Accidents	119	(1.9)	256	(22.6)	212	(36.1)	357	(44.0)	944	(10.7)
Cancer	37	(0.6)	105	(9.3)	137	(23.3)	141	(17.4)	420	(4.8)
Respiratory disease	429	(7.0)	106	(9.3)	25	(4.3)	28	(3.5)	588	(6.8)
Congenital anomalies	1,600	(26.1)	250	(22.0)	79	(13.4)	61	(7.5)	1,990	(22.9)
SIDS	1,165	(19.0)	30	(2.6)	–	—	–	—	1,195	(13.8)
All causes	6,141		1,135		588		811		8,675	

Table 1.3   Approximate number of cases of childhood cancer occurring each year in the current United Kingdom population of about 11 million children below aged 15 (From Draper and Stiller, 1989. Reproduced by kind permission of Scutari Projects Ltd)

	Male	Female	Total
Leukaemia	230	170	400
Lymphomas	90	40	130
Brain and spinal tumours	150	120	270
Embryonal tumours			
Wilms' tumour	35	35	70
Neuroblastoma	40	30	70
Retinoblastoma	20	20	40
Hepatoblastoma	5	5	10
Bone tumours	30	30	60
Soft tissue sarcomas	40	30	70
Other	30	40	70
Total	670	520	1,190

provides figures that are helpful in planning a service, but also offers an opportunity for research into both the causes of childhood cancer and its subsequent outcome.

WHAT CAUSES CHILDHOOD CANCER?

In spite of a great deal of research, there is still little known about the cause of most types of cancer in childhood. Certain chromosomal anomalies and other inherited conditions are associated with an increased risk of developing cancer in early life, and this supports the hypothesis that a genetic predisposition to cancer may underline many such cancers. The association of acute leukaemia with Down's syndrome is perhaps the best known. However, although there may be an underlying genetic predisposition in many children, this does not imply that childhood cancer is likely to recur in subsequent children in a family.

There are a few, rare types of cancer which *are* inherited and do occur in several members of one family and in subsequent generations. Retinoblastoma, a rare cancer of the eye, is the best-known example. The gene responsible for its inheritance has been localised to chromosome 13. It is likely that the specific chromosomes involved in many cancers will be identified over the next few years. In Wilms' tumour of the kidney there is often an abnormality of chromosome 11, while in Ewing's tumour of the bone another region of chromosome 11 is involved along with chromosome 22; and in neuroblastoma tumour of the sympathetic nervous system chromosome 1 appears to be involved.

The most popular theory as to the mechanism of causation of cancer in young people is the 'two-hit' hypothesis, first described by Knudson (1971). Knudson suggested that two 'insults' are required to cause cancer, the first often being while the baby is still in utero rendering it susceptible to the second 'hit' which can occur at any time thereafter. In the case of retinoblastoma the first hit might be the inheritance of an already abnormal gene, but for the majority of other cancers a mutation must take place early in foetal life leading to an abnormal gene which can subsequently be affected by the 'second hit'.

There have been many attempts to identify environmental factors which could be responsible for either of these 'hits'. Radiation is the best-known cause of leukaemia in childhood, yet it probably accounts for at most 5 per cent of all cases.

The evidence that radiation does cause leukaemia comes first from the observation of a high incidence of leukaemia in persons exposed to the two atomic bomb explosions in Japan in 1945 with a clear dose/response relationship – i.e. the closer the person to the bomb, the higher the dose of radiation received and, up to a certain level, the greater the risk of leukaemia. Secondly, it is now accepted that there is an increased risk of children developing leukaemia if their mothers had an abdominal X-ray during pregnancy, particularly in the first trimester. There are no other such clear associations between environmental factors and childhood cancer. Studies of the geographical distribution of cancer within countries have also been largely unrewarding but investigations of the patterns of cancer in different countries and different races has led to some clues, e.g. the association of Burkitt's lymphoma with the Epstein-Barr Virus (EBV) in the malaria belt of Africa. Ewing's tumour is virtually unknown in negro races, including in the United States, and this observation will no doubt eventually tell us something about the aetiology of this particular tumour, but at present the reason for this observation eludes us.

Following the diagnosis of cancer in their child the first response of most parents is 'What has caused it?' or 'Will it affect my other child?' If known familial conditions are excluded, e.g. retinoblastoma and neurofibromatosis – a condition characterised by developmental changes in the nervous system, muscles, bones and skin and marked by the formation of neurofibromas over the body associated with patches of pigmentation – then any sibling of a child with cancer will have approximately a 1:300 rather than 1:600 chance of also developing it during childhood. Most of the sibling pairs, however, are increasingly being recognised as belonging to 'cancer family syndromes', the best known of which is the Li-Fraumeni syndrome which consists of various tumours in siblings, e.g. rhabdomyosarcoma (a muscle tumour), adreno-cortical carcinoma and brain tumours along with breast cancer occurring at an early age in their mother. Behind the parents' question relating to causation often lies tremendous guilt feelings – 'Is it something that we have done, or not done?' The simple and reassuring answer to this is that, although we do not know what does cause cancer, we know an awful lot of things that do not and parents can be assured that it is nothing that they have done, either by commission or omission.

HOW DOES CANCER PRESENT IN CHILDREN?

The mode of presentation will depend on the type of cancer. Leukaemia is a disease of the bone marrow and presents with signs of bone marrow failure. Lack of red cells will give pallor and anaemia, thrombocytopenia or low platelets will lead to easy and extensive bruising, and the absence of normal white cells may give rise to infection. In addition, leukaemia cells can be found anywhere in the body but they have a special affinity for lymphatic tissues; consequently massive swelling of lymph nodes and enlargement of liver and spleen may be present. Solid tumours, on the other hand, may present in a variety of ways depending on the site and size of the primary tumour and whether or not there is any evidence of spread to other sites in the body.

This spread is known as metastatic disease and the secondary tumours are called metastases. A solid tumour will grow locally and may cause pain or symptoms due to pressure on surrounding structures. Cells may break off the primary tumour and spread to other parts of the body either via the blood or lymphatic channels. Even though it may not be possible to identify any metastases with the investigative measures that are available, we know that micrometastases are often present at diagnosis and it is for this reason that local treatment of a primary tumour, either by surgery and/or radiotherapy, is often insufficient to effect a cure. There are only a very few tumours, e.g. localised Hodgkin's disease, a disease of the lymphoid system, or some bone tumours which can be cured without systemic treatment.

INVESTIGATION OF A CHILD WITH CANCER

Many of the detailed investigations of a child with cancer are dealt with in subsequent chapters. Following the clinical suspicion that a child may have cancer the first procedures are directed towards making a positive diagnosis. In the vast majority of cases this will mean obtaining a specimen of tissue for laboratory investigation. For leukaemia the appropriate tissue will be bone marrow, although peripheral blood examined under the microscope will give an indication of the diagnosis. For solid tumours a piece of the tumour itself needs to be taken and sent to the laboratory for histological assessment. Many sophisticated techniques can now be applied to the investigation of cancer so that a classification into subtypes of any disease may be possible, e.g. leukaemia may be lymphoid or myeloid, depending on which white cells it is originating from, and lymphoid or lymphoblastic leukaemia can be subdivided into T cell, B cell, or common.

Occasionally it is not possible to obtain tissue for diagnosis because the tumour is inaccessible and surgery would be dangerous. Large tumours in the mediastinum and some in the brain have to be treated on the basis of a clinical and radiological diagnosis although whenever possible attempts are made to obtain a 'tissue diagnosis'.

Once the diagnosis has been made the next step is to 'stage' the tumour. Staging a tumour means delineating the extent of disease at the time of diagnosis and restaging may take place after treatment has been given. The stage of a tumour will depend on the site and size of the primary tumour and the presence (or not) of metastases. The staging system for Wilms' tumour (Figure 1.1) gives an example of such a system. In general, the more extensive the tumour, the higher the stage. Investigations are directed towards determining the size and relationships of the primary tumour and then the presence (or not) of metastases. Radiology, ultrasound and radioisotope

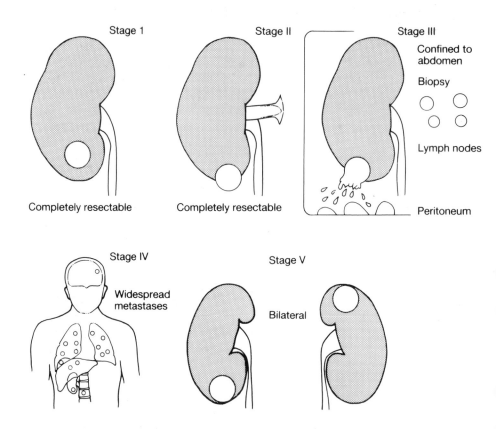

Figure 1.1.   Staging system used for Wilms' tumour (from Craft, 1981. Reproduced by kind permission of *Hospital Update*)

scans may all be necessary. For leukaemia, a stage is not usually given but the white cell count is usually taken as being equivalent to a stage.

What then is the purpose of such staging procedures? The prognosis or outcome for any particular disease is dependent on the stage at diagnosis. The more developed the stage the worse the prognosis usually is. Knowing the stage, therefore, enables an informed prognosis to be made. However, it also allows treatment to be given that is appropriate to the stage, more extensive tumours generally requiring more therapy with consequently less treatment being given to localised or lower stage disease. However, prognosis is not only dependent on the stage. Other prognostic factors may be important, e.g. age in leukaemia and histological subtype in other tumours.

OUTCOME OF CANCER IN CHILDREN

The prognosis for childhood cancer has improved quite dramatically over the past forty years and that in the last twenty years can be seen in Table 1.4. In the 1940–60 period a few children could be cured by surgery, sometimes with the addition of radiotherapy, but it was not until the advent of chemotherapy that the situation really began to improve. We have now reached the stage where between 60 and 70 per cent of all children diagnosed as having cancer can be cured. Being able to talk of *cure* itself is a dramatic change which twenty years ago we were very uncertain about. For some types of cancer the prognosis is extremely good, e.g. localised Wilms' tumour and Hodgkin's disease have cure rates of up to 90 per cent, although there are others, e.g. advanced neuroblastoma, where the outlook is still poor.

This improvement in survival has led to a change in the philosophy of treatment. Initially it was one of cure at almost 'any cost', but this has now changed to 'cure at least cost'. The reason is that with increasingly long survival, we are recognising that some treatments result in substantial long-term or 'late effects', although they have successfully cured the original cancer.

Table 1.4   Five-year percentage survival rates for principal types of childhood cancer diagnosed 1971–73 and 1980–82 (From Draper and Stiller, 1989. Reproduced by kind permission of Scutari Projects Ltd)

	Years of diagnosis	
	1971–73	1980–82
Acute lymphoblastic leukaemia	37	64
Acute non-lymphoblastic leukaemia	4	19
Hodgkin's disease	76	91
Non-Hodgkin's disease	21	55
Brain and spinal tumours	42	50
Neuroblastoma	16	35
Retinoblastoma	87	86
Wilms' tumour	58	75
Osteosarcoma	18	35
Ewing's tumour	37	33
Rhabdomyosarcoma	26	48
Malignant gonadal germ-cell tumours	50	84

It has become increasingly important to study these late effects. Among the more important are:

1.   Those due to radiotherapy, where the effect is dependent on the site to which the treatment was given, e.g.
   • Ovarian failure in patients treated for Wilms' tumour
   • Subtle intellectual damage in children with acute lympho-blastic leukaemia given cranial irradiation
   • Second primary malignancies within an irradiated area.

2.   Chemotherapy which can cause, e.g.
   • Infertility in boys given alkylating agents such as cyclo-phosphamide
   • Chronic renal insufficiency in those given cis-platinum.

This change in philosophy is perhaps best exemplified by Wilms' tumour where, in a series of carefully controlled studies, we have learnt that we can substantially limit treatment. In the 1960s and early 1970s early stage Wilms' tumour was treated by surgery, radiotherapy and by two and often more cytotoxic drugs. Most children survived but many of the girls are now infertile with ovarian failure. A child presenting in the United Kingdom (UK) now would receive surgery and a very short course of one drug. Hopefully, this will leave us with children who are, apparently, truly cured, i.e. no cancer and no late effects.

ORGANISATION OF CARE

The increasing complexity of treatments and the necessity for many different disciplines to be involved has led to the centralisation of care for children with cancer into specialised units. These have evolved over the last few years as their need has become apparent. However, this development has not been without some opposition. Families experience difficulties caused by geographical separation, and district general hospitals, which have to refer many of their interesting patients elsewhere, find consequent problems in staff morale, recruitment, retention and motivation.

If a referral for any illness is inevitable because a particular surgical skill or piece of equipment is only available in a regional centre, then this is more accepted, e.g. in the necessity for centralisation of care for cardiac and neurosurgery. However,

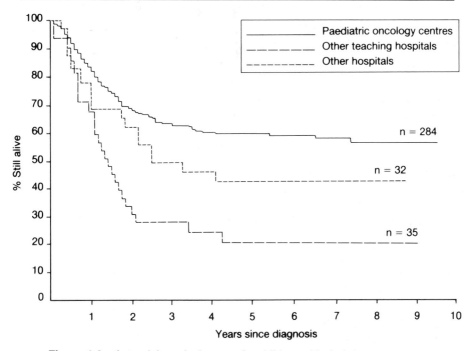

Figure 1.2   Actuarial survival curves for children with rhabdomyosarcoma classified by type of treatment centre (From Stiller, 1988. Reproduced by kind permission of the Department of Health)

with oncology the benefits to be achieved by specialist centres are more subtle, although there can be no doubt that it is in the child's best interests to be referred to a regional centre. Not only are the chances of survival substantially better for those who are referred but also the benefits of more modern and perhaps less mutilating therapy are available earlier. Figure 1.2 shows the dramatic benefits for survival for patients with rhabdomyosarcoma, a muscle tumour, who are referred to a specialist centre.

TEAM APPROACH

In caring for children with cancer, the prime object now is cure, with minimal physical, intellectual, psychological and social cost to both the children and their families. Thus the treatment and care of children with cancer demands a multidisciplinary approach involving medicine, nursing, social work, physiotherapy, dietetics, play therapy and teaching, and spans both the hospital and community services. The senior nurse on a children's cancer unit has many individuals and departments to relate to. Some of these are shown in Figure 1.3.

NURSING THE CHILD WITH CANCER

Nursing plays a major contribution in the care and support of families affected by childhood cancer. In order to ensure that patients receive optimal care nurses must have a clear perspective of their role, the problems which they can help to alleviate or even mitigate, and the range of interventions available to them.

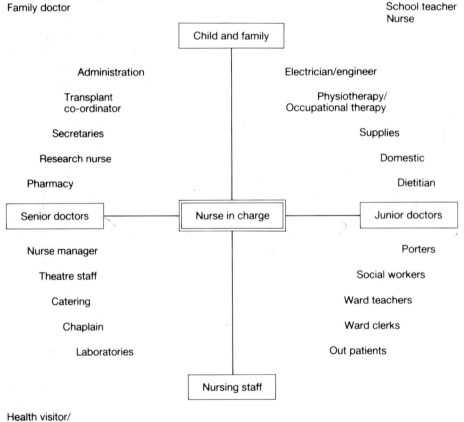

Figure 1.3   People with whom the nurse in charge interrelates

ROLE OF THE NURSE

Virginia Henderson (1966) has defined three roles of the nurse:

- a dependent function whereby the nurse carries out the doctor's prescribed treatment, assisting with procedures, e.g. administration of chemotherapy
- an interdependent function whereby the nurse plays a key role in coordinating services provided for the patients (Figure 1.3)
- an independent function which involves assisting, as appropriate, patients with their normal self-caring activities.

NURSING PROBLEMS OF CHILD WITH CANCER

There is a wide range of problems potentially amenable to nursing intervention which commonly affect children with cancer, i.e. those related to

- the disease itself
- the side-effects of treatment
- the psychosocial aspects of a long-term, potentially fatal illness requiring frequent periods of hospitalisation and/or intensive treatment
- for some, the terminal stages of the disease.

The nurse therefore, in order to plan appropriate nursing care, requires a knowledge of normal physiology, child development and the needs of children and their families, and the effect of the disease on normal functioning. The potential side-effects of treatment, as well as a good understanding of the emotional impact of loss and grief and ways in which it can be either alleviated or prevented, are particularly important in paediatric oncology.

In order to identify accurately the problems and potential problems for individual children and their families the nurse should adopt a systematic approach to assessment. This may be based on a recognised model of nursing, e.g. Henderson (1966), Roper, Logan and Tierney (1980), Roy (1980) or Orem (1971). Whichever model is adopted, it should include physical, psychological and emotional factors.

Nursing Intervention

When providing nursing care for children, nursing intervention is often more appropriately given indirectly through the parents rather than directly to the children themselves. This arguably constitutes the greatest difference between nursing children and nursing adults and is the reason why a family-centred approach to nursing has been more widely practised in paediatric settings than in adult services.

While in the past there has been a tendency for nurses to emphasise in their practice the giving of direct physical care, nurses are now more conscious of other ways in which they can contribute to patient care in a more positive way. Orem (1971) indentified these other helping strategies as:

- guiding
- supporting, both physically and psychologically
- providing an environment that promotes personal development
- teaching.

In working with children with cancer and their families, paediatric nurses are increasingly expanding their use of these strategies. For example:

- Teaching parents to manage intravenous central lines and enteral feeding at home.
- With other members of the team providing teaching packages/programmes for children and families, who with greater knowledge and understanding of the disease and treatment gain a more positive feeling of being in control of their lives, all of which allows them to contribute more fully in decision-making.
- Appropriate use of listening and counselling skills enable children and families to cope more positively with the psychosocial impact of loss and grief.

ORGANISATION OF NURSING SERVICES

The nursing of children with cancer readily lends itself to primary nursing, in which a specific nurse is identified as having responsibility for the assessment, planning, implementation and evaluation of the nursing care for individual children and their families. This provides the families with one person whom they can identify as their link person and questions can be channelled through the nurse to others who may need to provide more information or clarification on that already given. Many centres are now developing nurses with special skills in, for example, bone marrow transplantation, home care, etc. It is important to recognise that the larger the paediatric oncology unit becomes, the more difficult is communication. Full documentation of all encounters with children and their families is essential and a system needs to be identified for the dissemination of this information to those who need to know.

As the nurse's role develops, areas of interdisciplinary conflict can arise, e.g. there is a 'grey area' between nursing and social work in terms of 'counselling' children and families. Nurses should not adopt roles for which they are untrained but where they do have special skills 'the team' must find a way of allowing these to be used for the benefit of the patient. Paediatric oncology nursing is an emotionally enormously demanding speciality but this is amply offset by the rewards of seeing children with a potentially fatal disease grow into healthy adults.

References

Court D (1976) *Fit for the Future: Report of the Committee on Child Health Services.* London: HMSO.

Craft A (1981) *Hospital Update*, Jan: 13.

Draper G and Stiller C (1989) Cautious optimism. *Paediatric Nursing*, **1**(3): 22–24.

Henderson V (1966) *The Nature of Nursing.* London: Collier Macmillan.

Knudson A G (1971) *Mutation and Cancer Statistical Study Retinoblastoma Proceedings at the National Academy of Science USA*, **68**: 820–823.

Orem D E (1971) *Nursing Concepts of Practice.* New York: McGraw-Hill.

Roper N, Logan W W and Tierney A J (1980) *The Elements of Nursing.* London: Churchill Livingstone.

Roy C (1980) Adaptation model. In: Riehl J P and Roy C (eds.), *Conceptual Models for Nursing Practice*, 2nd edition. New York: Appleton-Century-Crofts.

Stiller C (1988) Centralisation of treatment and survival rates for cancer. *Archives of Disease in Childhood*, **63**: 26.

Further Reading

Court D and Alberman E (1988) Worlds apart. In: *Child Health in a Changing Society*. London: Oxford University Press.

Stiller C A (1988) Centralisation of treatment and survival rates for cancer, *Archives of Disease in Childhood*, **63:** 23.

Stiller C A and Draper G J (1989) Treatment centre size, Entry to trials and survival in acute lymphoblastic leukaemia, *Archives of Disease in Childhood*, **64:** 657.

2
The Family of the Child with Cancer

- The three weeks in hospital were like being in another world – in fact, for me, life outside the hospital ceased to exist. It was almost as if Sarah and I became a single person – we grew so close, physically and emotionally.*

This is a statement from the mother of a three-year-old, newly diagnosed as having leukaemia. It shows something of the intensity of the relationship between parent and child, so often experienced when a child is diagnosed as having a life-threatening illness.

THE FAMILY

Children are a part of a family unit, but what is 'the family'? The family is the significant group of people who are the child's primary support group in his life, e.g. parent, foster parent, guardian, siblings or others (RCN, 1986). Therefore, according to this definition, any family unit that nursing staff may encounter will probably differ from child to child. Each will be a family unit in its own right and, usually, is the place where the child feels most secure.

The vast majority of children receiving hospital treatment will have at least one parent either resident or visiting frequently. For this reason, throughout this chapter, I shall refer to the family as involving parents.

Relevance of Family Factors to the Child with Cancer

Jennings (1986) states that only in recent years have families been recognised for their significant role in the care of their children in hospital.

The reactions of a child to his illness and changing situation/environment will be dependent on many factors, particularly on those that relate to his family. It is important, then, that we consider family factors when planning the care of the child with cancer.

Parental Influence

Children depend on their parents (or surrogate) for physical care, psychological and emotional welfare, education and social training. When a child becomes ill, some of these functions may be taken on, of necessity, by other people. The way in which the child is used to being handled, spoken to and involved by his parents, in family situations, will be largely responsible for his response to other people.

Parents may feel that their influence over their child, newly diagnosed with cancer, has diminished and therefore cease to behave towards him in their usual way. It is important for nursing staff, from the very beginning of their relationship with families, to encourage parents to be involved in the care of their child as much as they want. At this early stage in the nurse/family relationship, the parents may feel unable to participate as fully as when the relationship progresses.

The Child's Position in the Family

The size of the family, and the child's relationship with siblings, will also have an impact on the child in his day-to-day life and therefore will be another factor in determining his reactions to his new situation. For example, in a small family more emphasis is placed on individual development of the children and there is more in the way of pressure on the child to measure up to family expectations. In a large family, children are more likely to be able to adjust to changes and crises, as there is more emphasis on the group than on the individual (Whaley and Wong, 1985). We can observe this in children in hospital or undergoing prolonged treatment.

A child's position in the family will affect his view of the world and his relationships with others. Whaley and Wong state: 'In general, the narrower the spacing between siblings, the more the children influence each other. The wider the spacing, the greater the influence of the parents.'

Siblings

Having a child with cancer in the family may result in the parents and other adult members focusing all their attention on

the sick child. As a result, there may be problems with siblings
who feel left out, unwanted and unloved. If older, they may
also feel guilty that it is not they who are sick or even wish to
change places with the sick sibling. One mother wrote, of her
nine-year-old son: 'Peter experienced feelings of jealousy,
aggression and great unhappiness during Andrew's [age 5]
illness. He looked for support through the hospital and the
church.'

Honesty with siblings, and allowing them to be involved in
the care of the sick child, generally leads to greater trust in the
parents and professional carers. Promoting this feeling of worth
appears to make problems easier to deal with, either when the
sick child has recovered or died. Jennings (1986) emphasises
that siblings benefit from being with their family, resolving the
strain of separation and some of the fantasies built up about the
hospitalised child.

A mother reported of her ten-year-old son, following the
death of his six-year-old brother, that, because of his anger and
the difficulties they were experiencing in communicating with
him at home, a child guidance counsellor proved very helpful.
During this therapy it was discovered that he was experiencing
many of the feelings of loss he had experienced when his
parents divorced six years earlier and had never expressed.

Siblings can be of great importance to a sick child (Figure 2.1).

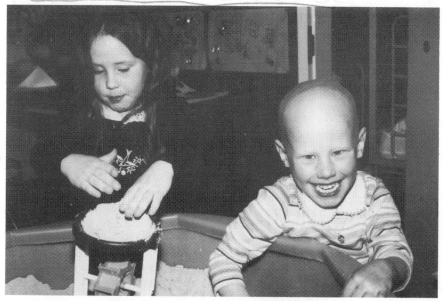

Figure 2.1   A sibling joins her brother in play

One mother of a nine-year-old, with acute lymphoblastic leukaemia, wrote, 'His younger brother was the first person he wanted to see when admitted to hospital.'

Ways in which the Family May Cope

This is an important factor in the care of the child with cancer. The sick child, who will probably have become the centre of everybody's attention, will:

- probably mirror certain of the ways in which he sees his parents coping, and
- react to his condition and treatment according to the way he sees his parents and other family members coping.

Ways in which family members cope in response to this situation may or may not have been experienced by them in previous situations. Individuals may have difficulty in accepting the way they themselves, or other members of the family, are coping with a child with cancer and the implications of the diagnosis and treatment.

One of the most important and common ways individuals have of coping with a difficult situation is to talk. Nursing staff ideally need to be available at any time to enable members of the child's family to do this. This is a very supportive nursing role and may not require the nurse to do much talking herself, but to listen. Parents may have difficulty putting their true feelings into words. Nurses need to develop special skills in listening to what is *not* being said. This will, in some circumstances, encourage families to voice their real feelings and fears.

Some individuals may need a period, or regular periods, of silence or solitude in order to cope with aspects of their child's illness and/or treatment.

- Nurses must be prepared to accept parental reactions and defences – anger, hostility, rejection, dependency – without anger and without withdrawing themselves from the situation. (Whaley and Wong, 1985).

Nurses are very much needed for many families as a help, comfort and support. They in turn need to feel well supported in order to fulfil this very demanding role.

The Extended Family

The family, as described before, may be extended – to grandparents, aunts, uncles, cousins, and so on. The extent to which these family members may be involved in the care of a sick or hospitalised child is often determined by culture. For example, Asian families are more likely to have grandparents, aunts and uncles involved in caring for the child. In the United Kingdom, people are more mobile than they used to be, and so families are likely to be dispersed throughout the country or even live overseas. Members of the extended family may often find difficulty in visiting or offering practical help on a regular basis.

Grandparents generally need particular consideration. They are not only agonising over the diagnosis of cancer and its effect on their grandchild, but have to bear the additional stress of watching their own child dealing with such a painful situation.

Members of the extended family may want to become involved immediately in the care of the sick child, to the exclusion of all else. Skilful counselling will enable them to realise their potential as a real support to the parents. This support may take the form of caring for siblings, providing meals, or acting as a 'messenger' in relating progress reports to anxious friends and relatives. They may also be able to provide a respite for a resident parent to go home for a bath, some sleep or to spend time with other children, away from the hospital environment.

EFFECTS OF DIAGNOSIS

The family who have just been told that their child has cancer will be devastated and, quite likely, in a state of shock for a variable period of time. They are often unable to take in all that is being said to them while in this state.

Whaley and Wong explain that 'Because a family is a system of interdependent parts, a change in any one member of the system causes a corresponding change in every other member.'

In many instances, the reactions of parents will be similar. Whaley and Wong state that initially *denial and disbelief* may be experienced. *Guilt and/or anger* may be the next reaction experienced, guilt being an almost universal response. *Fear, anxiety and frustration* are all common reactions to the realisation that one's child has a potentially fatal disease.

In response to the question 'Can you remember your immediate reaction/feeling after being told of Andrew's diagnosis?' Andrew's parents wrote:

- It was like having a terrifying nightmare that you woke up from and found was true. Our physical reaction was one of shock, feeling weak at the knees, shaky, etc., and of disbelief. We also felt guilty.

    I remember experiencing the same reaction, but this time twice as hard, when I was told months later that Andrew was likely to die. This time I was told in a corridor by the two doctors on the ward. After they left me I remember wandering around with a wobbly feeling in my legs and a dazed feeling in my head. I felt as if I had been hit with a sledge hammer. My husband was not with me, so I had no one to hang on to. I remember telling parents I vaguely knew what I had just been told. I think that was my worst moment.

Fear, devastation, desolation, desperation, relief and un-certainty are reactions described by other parents when asked the same question. The effects of the diagnosis of childhood cancer will change for each family with ongoing treatment and results. Parents will often grieve for the 'normal' child they have lost in a similar way to grieving after somebody has died. The attitude of family members to the sick child is likely to change permanently because of this process. It can be seen from the reactions described above how important it is to choose the right time and place to tell parents any devastating news. It is usually helpful for them to be together, not only for initial support, but for interpretation of the news.

Another dilemma which parents face is what or how to tell the sick child. This will largely be determined by the child's age and level of understanding. A most common initial reaction is that parents do not want their child to know that he has cancer. In time, they will often change their minds about this. Nurses need to be there if parents need education, support and guidance in this area.

Whaley and Wong state, 'Siblings' reactions to a sister's or brother's illness or hospitalisation are anger, resentment, jealousy and guilt.' The amount of information siblings will be given about a brother's or sister's diagnosis will depend on their age, maturity, family discussion systems and how parents are able to come to terms with it themselves. Effects of a diagnosis of childhood cancer will be far-reaching, affecting not only the immediate and extended family. School friends, neighbours, godparents and casual acquaintances will all, in some way, be affected by this diagnosis. The effect it has on people outside the family will largely determine their reaction towards the family of the ill child. The family may have to make the first move in conversation, mentioning cancer, its treatment and side-effects.

FAMILY-CENTRED CARE

Since families have assumed much more significance in the care of sick children, family-centred care has become very important. 'The goal of family-centred care is to maintain or strengthen the roles and ties of the family, with the hospitalised child, in order to promote normality of the family unit' (Brunner and Suddarth, 1978). The family should be encouraged to be involved in the planning and implementing of the care of their child, under nursing supervision, while he is in hospital.

Bivalec and Berkman (1976) believe that parents can become responsible participants in all phases of care, provided they are willing to do so. The amount of involvement will vary from family to family, and nursing staff should be available to advise and support the family in this role. For many families, this will be something they had not anticipated. Some families will wish to be involved in all aspects of their child's care – technical, emotional and developmental. Others will wish to avoid the technical side of caring, leaving that to the nursing staff. Families need to be educated in different aspects of their child's care, thus enabling them to decide the extent of their own involvement.

Geen (1986) states that 'The child with cancer is likely to need several periods of hospitalisation, many outpatients visits and prolonged contact with the hospital.' He may also require prolonged treatment. Explanations of treatment and side-effects to the family will increase their understanding and help them to feel more in control of what is happening to their child. These explanations need to be directed appropriately, depending on the family's individual needs and understanding.

Another way in which families are able to feel more relaxed and involved is by the introduction of a primary nurse (Figure 2.2). Geen explains:

- To a child his primary nurse is his 'special' nurse. She is the one with whom he builds up a trusting and secure relationship for the duration of his hospital stay. The primary nurse is responsible for the assessment, planning, documentation, implementation and evaluation of the 24-hour care of her patients wherever possible.

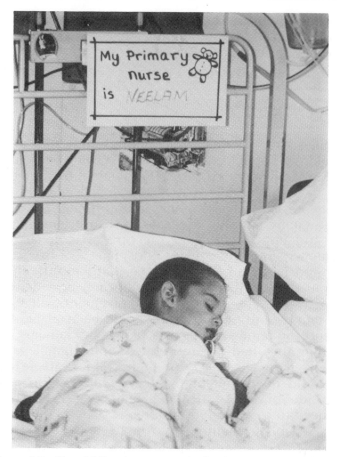

Figure 2.2   The child's primary nurse is clearly named at the bedside

If the child develops a particular trusting relationship with one nurse, and she involves the family too, the family feel they have a central figure to turn to for information, talk things over with and, if necessary, deliver criticism to.

RELIGIOUS AND CULTURAL NEEDS

We live in a multi-cultural society, and it is important to understand and respect different cultures and religions as part of our job in caring effectively for children with cancer. These factors have a great influence on many families and religion in particular may be a great source of comfort and support.

Culturally, some families will wish to have many more

members involved in the care of their child. For other families, much greater restriction will be practised.

Families may come from abroad to have their child's condition treated. This may present communication problems in the form of a language barrier. Interpreters are vital in this situation and a list of willing people is a useful addition to a ward notice board.

- An interpreter helped the nurses understand this family's cultural needs, which were not being met by the environment. The noise level, large number of people and lack of privacy, contributed to the mother's stress. (Jennings, 1986).

Certain cultures and religions also have dietary requirements. It is essential to ascertain these quickly and to enquire if the hospital catering can meet these needs. If the hospital is unable to supply a particular diet, nursing staff need to help parents to make alternative arrangements for their child's diet.

Although we live in a nominally Christian country, we are often ignorant of needs within our own Christian faith, as well as those of other religions. Because of our ignorance, we are often guilty of ignoring the spiritual needs of children and their families, unless prompted by the families to do so. Spiritual needs often surface suddenly when the family is faced with a devastating situation, such as life-threatening disease. These needs are often difficult to recognise in children, but are more obviously present in their parents. Shelly (1982) says in her book about the spititual needs of children, 'Each child is unique. Each comes from a different family background, a particular religious upbringing and a unique set of life experiences. Each child stands at his or her own special place in spiritual development.' Shelly explains that the primary burden of responsibility for the spiritual care of children lies with parents. She says that, as good nursing care sees children as part of a family network, spiritual care should do the same.

Hospital chaplains, layworkers and clergy from local churches play a very important part in the spiritual care and development of sick children and their families. Often, when distressed, parents are quite happy to talk about spiritual matters with people who do not share the same religious faith.

Some religions, particularly Eastern religions, require special facilities or particularly quiet places for their prayer times. It is very helpful if staff can be aware of this and meet needs wherever possible.

One family have expressed their great fortune in receiving

three kinds of support when their five-year-old son was sick and dying:

- *Practical* from hospital staff, friends and neighbours.
- *Emotional* from hospital staff, other parents and friends.
- *Spiritual* from the church, which 'grew as Stephen's illness progressed and, at his death, became our greatest source of support.'

THOUGHTS FROM SOME FAMILIES

Many parents find it a great help to verbalise or write down their feelings and thoughts about various aspects of their child's illness, treatment and, if appropriate, death. Soon after the diagnosis of leukaemia in her three-year-old daughter, a mother said that she found it impossible to leave Sarah with anyone other than her husband. The parents of the same little girl wrote:

- We both made a conscious effort to say, 'this is the situation, we have no control over it and, shattered/desperate as we are, the sooner we accept the situation, the sooner we can begin to re-organise our lives around it.' Once we had come to terms with things in this way which wasn't easy we could begin, on a day-to-day basis, to build for the future we weren't sure whether Sarah had.

Families become very dependent on the hospital staff. The mother of a five-year-old boy who had just completed his first course of treatment for abdominal lymphoma said:

- I remember, after a week's treatment in hospital, we were told we could go home for a while. I did not feel we were ready to go home. It was like being abandoned. I felt quite dependent on the hospital, but was not yet sure who to trust. Other feelings, at this time, were of anger, fear and still disbelief that this was happening to us.

On being asked if she and her husband felt as involved as they wanted to be with their son's care, the mother wrote:

- We were encouraged to look after our child as much as possible and take on responsibility for all his needs, except the giving of drugs. Andrew was also very involved and liked to give injections via a central venous catheter himself and to choose the order he wanted his drugs in. On occasions, if I felt tired or a bit depressed, it would have been nice for a nurse to have taken over for a while. However, staff shortages kept the nurses very busy.

This shows how important it is for parents to be able to hand over the care of their child periodically. It also shows how, very often, parents will be sympathetic towards the demands put on professional carers.

On answering the same question the mother of a two-year-old, being treated for testicular rhabdomyosarcoma, wrote:

- I did feel, however unjustified, that I had no control over various drugs that were being administered. The system appeared, to me anyway, rather like a machine that would continue regardless, and if I did question anything, I felt as if I was being distrustful.

This same mother has since said that these were her feelings at the time of Hugo's treatment and that she was not ungrateful.

Parents have indicated that nursing staff play a very important part in caring for their sick child and his family. The following thoughts have been expressed:

- It is comforting to think we can talk to the hospital staff and individual nurses who, we hope, are friends now, as well as being skilled nurses.

- The nursing staff were superb – extremely supportive, sympathetic, understanding and incredibly patient. They were never too busy to talk or reassure.

- Andrew formed strong attachments to some of the nurses and was always much happier when his favourite was on duty. He would spend a lot of time following nurses around, trying to 'help' them. His favourite nurse always came and said goodbye when going off duty.

Most families appear to feel that they are given adequate information concerning drugs, treatment and side-effects. Many like to have information written down.

It appears that many parents have some idea of the diagnosis of cancer before it is confirmed by medical personnel. This thought is usually pushed to the back of their minds because, as one parent writes, 'I never thought it could affect our child. Diseases like leukaemia only affect someone else's children – don't they?'

The family of Sarah, the three-year-old with acute lympho-blastic leukaemia, said that they were impressed with the way they were told of her diagnosis by their family doctor. They also said that they would have appreciated more reassurance from him. At the same time they realised that their GP was unable to give this reassurance because he had 'never dealt with a child with leukaemia before'. This is a common problem, as most GPs will only come across one or two cases of childhood cancer in their practising lifetime. Also, the signs and symptoms of childhood cancer may resemble other childhood illnesses. Parents may, therefore, have taken their child to the surgery on several occasions before a diagnosis is finally made.

Outpatient Visits

Parents see outpatient visits as an opportunity:

- to receive confirmation of their child's continuing satisfactory progress,
- to bring any anxieties to the attention of medical staff, and
- to discuss further treatment.

The week leading up to an outpatient visit is often an anxious time for parents as they contemplate what may be said and, often, may be particularly concerned at the possibility of receiving bad news.

Parents express a need for outpatient visits as a continuation of inpatient care or for ongoing treatment but frequently complain about waiting times – a common problem wherever they are treated. This waiting time can be used to good effect by talking to staff and other families, although often stress prevents a relaxed conversation. As one parent commented: 'Although one is naturally sympathetic about other children's illnesses, one is more concerned about one's own child's status.'
Another parent commented:

- One of the advantages of attending the outpatient clinic was seeing children who have been 'cured' returning for their check-ups. This was important because we were generally used to seeing ill children or hearing of those who were dying.

Parents often feel confused after waiting a long time to see the doctor and forget to ask questions that had been in their mind. A way of overcoming this problem is to encourage parents to write down their questions and to look at what they have written during consultation.

Children often look upon outpatient visits as a time to see old friends, play with other children and somebody else's toys. It can be a time of anxiety for them too, worrying about future unpleasant treatments or remembering previous ones.

OTHER INFLUENCES

There are usually many people involved in supporting and caring for families of children with cancer. The hospital nurse may not come into direct contact with these people. They include family, friends, neighbours, school teachers, school nurses, health visitors, family doctors and clergy. They may each play a very important role in caring for the families when they are at home, or taking care of things at home while the sick child is in hospital.

Reactions of family and friends to diagnosis and treatment, side-effects and their implications are important to the sick child and his family. One mother said: 'Many people looked for our reaction before expressing their feelings'; and another:

- There is a tendency amongst our family and friends to treat Hugo differently. We did not, however, over-react or seek sympathy, which may have prevented the situation from becoming too dramatic. It also helped life carry on as normally as possible.

Support

Many parents have said that their greatest support during their child's illness has come from each other. It is important to encourage this, if possible, to help parents communicate with each other.

Social services will also have a large part to play with some families. There may be financial or travel difficulties and the hospital social worker can be an invaluable source of support and help.

Families of children with cancer find great support from hospital staff. Compassionate and consistent carers give tremendous support and often make children feel safe and secure.

Parents of children with cancer can offer support to each other, they often build up long-term relationships and there is an empathy between them that nobody else can share.

The child with cancer will receive greater support from his family if they too are well supported. Peers can offer much support, even if unknowingly. Visits from school friends are often much longed for. Letters and cards from school or cubs/ brownies or other organisations are a source of great pleasure to a sick child. It is not always easy for the parents of these young friends to feel happy about their offspring visiting a friend with cancer. They worry about their child's reaction to hair loss and vomiting, drugs and tubes. They may worry about the questions they themselves will have to face, and the implications of their answers – perhaps questions about the death of a child or implications of the disease. The mother of a five-year-old with lymphoma wrote:

- Stephen had school friends who were brave enough to visit him. He was not always in the mood for seeing them, but felt reassured by their attention. Some parents of Stephen's friends were rather cautious about their own child's reaction to seeing Stephen and other children at the hospital, being naturally worried that they might be distressed.

Some families will have more support from outside the hospital than others. The family who have recently moved to the area or even to this country may need all their support from hospital staff and from each other. The parents of a two-year-old wrote: 'We received great support from our child, and his determination to have a normal childhood, even when undergoing treatment.'

References

Bivalec L M and Berkman J (1976) *Care of Parents.* The Nursing Clinics of North America. Philadelphia: W B Saunders.

Brunner L S and Suddarth D S (1978) *The Lippincott Manual of Paediatric Nursing.* London: Harper and Row.

Geen L J (1986) A special friend. *Nursing Times/Nursing Mirror,* **82**(36): 32–33.

Jennings K (1986) Helping them face tomorrow. *Nursing Times,* **22**(4): 33–35.

RCN Society of Paediatric Nursing (1986) Statement of values in paediatric nursing, *Newsletter No. 11.* London: RCN.

Shelly A J et al (1982) *Spiritual Needs of Children.* Intervarsity Christian Fellowship of USA: 67.

Whaley L F and Wong D L (1985) *Essentials of Paediatric Nursing,* 2nd edition. St Louis: C V Mosby.

Note:

*Quotations from parents taken from answers to an informal questionnaire distributed, by myself, to five families.

3

Common Issues Relating to Diagnosis and Treatment

Many of the problems, both physical and psychosocial, are common to most children with cancer. It is a disease with far-reaching effects throughout the whole family: their lives will never be quite the same again whether the outcome for their child is cure or premature death.

PSYCHOSOCIAL EFFECTS

The Family

As most children are treated in one of the twenty children's cancer centres throughout the United Kingdom the family is frequently separated during the treatment period. The mother often stays with the child receiving treatment while the rest of the family are at home. Siblings may be looked after by relatives or friends while the father carries on with his job.

Family separation causes stress to all family members. The mother with the sick child can be up day and night giving much of the physical care, and is the first to receive all news, both good and bad. Father tries to keep up with work which has its own pressures and to keep the family home running smoothly, the bills paid and the house cleaned.

Siblings may be at home or staying with friends or relatives. If they are away from home parents have to find time to spend with them together as a family, and together as a couple. Separation creates division within any family; the parent staying with the sick child may feel tired, strained and alone with little privacy, while the parent at home may feel distant, isolated and equally alone. Siblings may be confused and feel rejected by their parents. Careful explanation by parents and reinforcement by those with whom brothers/sisters are staying may help, but family stress and separation is commonplace.

The provision of a place within the hospital complex for the family to be together is essential, preferably comfortable residential accommodation in a non-clinical environment yet near the ward. A room where all family members may be resident with adequate facilities and privacy in relaxed surroundings is ideal. If possible the ill child should join the family for some of the time. In practice, this arrangement is often only feasible in centres where the physical environment allows this.

REPEATED HOSPITALISATION

The amount of time spent in hospital is determined by the type of cancer the child has and the subsequent treatment programme.

The more readily curable childhood cancers such as Stage I or II Wilms' tumour (nephroblastoma) or Hodgkin's disease require mostly outpatient care following investigation and diagnosis. More resistant diseases such as acute myeloid leukaemia and Stage IV neuroblastoma require repeated and prolonged hospital care.

The period of waiting between the preliminary diagnosis, investigation, staging and the commencement of treatment is very traumatic for the child and his family. A period of high anxiety, anger and fear is followed by adjustment and in time acceptance of the situation. Families need to know what confronts them and an open and honest discussion, along with written details of the planned treatment, must always be given. All such discussions with the family should involve a nurse, as nursing staff are in a position actively to support the child and his family. It is acknowledged that parents and families do not hear or comprehend all that is being said to them during the initial interview with medical staff. The nurse is able, following the interview, to answer questions and clarify information given about the diagnosis and treatment plans. Following discussion with the family and child, the nurse is able to document what the child and family have been told in the nursing care plan. The child (if appropriate, depending upon age and understanding) and the parents should have access to and participate in this documentation.

Relationships with staff members and with other parents on the unit are important to many families. Some may last only for the duration of the child's illness but some go on much longer. Though important, these relationships are demanding and can become a great commitment for the nurse or other parents. A dependence on the unit, both the physical space and the people in it, can be a great relief and a great burden. It is a relief during treatment but towards the end that dependence can easily become a burden as families realise they are about to go home and not to return. Reassurance of staff still being there to help and support, along with written instructions giving names and telephone numbers and a promise of home visits, can help in the transition from hospital to home.

PHYSICAL EFFECTS — *impact of child*

Normality/Development

Childhood development depends to a great extent upon the physical, emotional and social world in which the child lives. The diagnosis of cancer with repeated hospitalisation, loss of schooling and reduced contact with peer groups will affect development. Setbacks in early childhood are difficult to remedy; therefore, all carers must endeavour to create an environment in hospital to encourage near normal activity.

Play specialists and teachers are important members of the team, as they get to know the child well and develop close relationships with families. Play involves enjoyment, relief from boredom, amusement and a degree of normality even for very sick children. With the expertise of the play specialist parents can be encouraged to help their children cope with their own illnesses. Through play the child is often able to express his feelings which he is unable to do in words. Play facilities are essential as a child's development is assisted through play, be it planned therapeutic play by health carers or spontaneous play by the child.

The playroom should be seen as the child's sanctuary, a place where they are free from clinical activities. Unpleasant procedures such as blood sampling should not take place in *their* room. Nursing and medical staff should go into the playroom to talk and play with the children, thus breaking down barriers of fear and demonstrating to the child that they are real people too.

Popular games are often associated with hospital activities. Through play children can inflict procedures such as finger pricks, bone marrow aspirations, the siting of infusions and changes of dressings on their dolls and teddies and even pretend with each other, their parents or staff. Other popular playroom activities include music-making, cooking and water play. Children readily adapt to playing with one free arm when the other arm is attached to an intravenous infusion (IVI). For this reason extension lines on the IVI should be routine to allow maximum flexibility and the infusion should preferably be sited in the less used limb. Playrooms also need multiple electric sockets to enable intravenous pumps to be plugged in. It is very frustrating to a child to have to leave the playroom in order that his pump battery be recharged in the middle of an important play session.

Not all children have access to the playroom and those nursed in isolation rooms and the older child or adolescent also need attention. Televisions and videos are important sources of contact for them, especially video films of home life to help keep them in touch. The adolescent is not always well catered for. An adolescent recreation room is the ideal (see also Chapter 9).

Projects, books and games are adaptable to time spent in isolation. Regular time set aside between the parent and the play specialist can give a lot of enjoyment to the child, as well as structure to the day. Keeping up with school work may be difficult. Experienced hospital teachers achieve good results by liaising with the child's own school and planning educational activities with the parents. They encourage active involvement for short periods at regular intervals in order not to overtire their pupils. On discharge from hospital or between treatments hospital teachers will refer work back to the child's own school or their personal tutor.

One problem often not anticipated by the family is treating the child as normal. Treating him as a chronic invalid, 'wrapping him in cotton wool', not allowing him to play with children outside the family in case he picks up an infection or is teased are all commonplace. Talking about the sick child as though he is not there, spoiling or prematurely mourning him are frequent strategies adopted by families where a child has cancer. Awareness of these phenomena by carers may prevent problems occurring, but most parents need help and guidance from nurses, social workers, doctors or psychologists to help them to cope with reverting to 'normal'. Talking freely about the disease and the implications of treatment within the family and the local community helps. If it is not talked about misconceptions are more likely to occur. Abnormal behaviours such as depression, regression and temper tantrums are less likely to occur and less difficult to address in an open and honest environment.

BODY IMAGE

Prolonged illness causes outward signs for all to see. Aggressive cancer treatments where the malignancy must be eradicated to preserve life has its effects on all tissues, and not just those affected by the disease. All rapidly dividing cells are affected by chemotherapy – the hair, gut, skin and the nail tissue deteriorate. This leads to a change in physical appearance and an alteration, often only temporary, in body image. If part of the treatment consists of radical disfiguring surgery, such as amputation for the removal of an osteosarcoma (bone tumour), and side-effects such as those following total body irradiation, this will effect permanent change both physical and psychological.

We are all affected by changes to our body image but it may be argued that younger children are less affected by weight or hair loss, poor skin structure and scarring than older children. However, many young children will grow up and may have to face problems later.

Radiotherapy can appear to have few effects on the small child but as he grows, areas that have been treated may grow less well and may lead to asymmetry of the body. Limbs and joints especially often fail to develop properly if irradiated for a cancer such as rhabdomyosarcoma (a muscle tumour) or for an osteosarcoma. Soft tissues such as the breast may fail to develop if one side of the chest is irradiated and not the other. Irradiation of the spine will lead to poor or distorted growth.

These are all well-recognised problems following treatment for childhood cancer and a much greater awareness of the problems has reduced long-term effects. Short-term changes during and immediately after treatment are unavoidable. Virtually all systemic chemotherapy results in hair loss. Although it cannot be avoided, coping with it by preparing the child helps. Even small children are bewildered when their hair begins to fall out, and are mostly concerned about hair getting in their mouth or in the bed. Making sure that their bed is kept hair-free and perhaps wearing a paper cap to catch the hair can help. Arrangements for alternative head cover can be discussed and organised in advance. Many children do not seem to want to cover their heads while in the ward but may refuse to go out of the hospital for a walk or refuse visitors because of it. Hats –

e.g. American baseball caps – of the latest fashion, scarves and wigs are all useful depending on personal choice. The use of dolls whose hair can be removed may help smaller children to understand what is happening. Not only should the child be helped to understand that there will be hair loss but also that the hair will grow back.

Body image can also be altered by the insertion of a tunnelled central venous catheter (e.g. Hickman or Broviac). Catheters are usually in situ for the duration of treatment. They are an important aid to treatment and improve the quality of life in many patients once the addition to the body is accepted. If the child is old enough to care for his catheter himself, acceptance is greater. Many become very attached to their catheter and want to keep it after it is removed. Again diagrams, drawings and booklets explaining what the catheter is for and how it functions assist the child to understand its placement.

Amputation of a limb for osteosarcoma has always been a cause of distress for patients with cancer. Physically, young children seem to adapt well though the acceptance by those around them may not be so positive. With modern surgery the preservation of a limb by replacing the affected bone with a telescopic prosthesis to grow with the child has become possible. It retains an aesthetically pleasing result and a functional limb. In the past it was thought that there was little point in retaining a non-functioning limb as children usually adapt well to their prosthestic limbs with little loss of function.

Tumour regrowth, particularly rhabdomyosarcoma of the head and neck, causes unsightly and distressing problems. Palliative radiotherapy may prevent further outward destruction in this very difficult situation.

The psychological effects of having cancer alone may create a poor body image and reduce self-esteem. Depression and loneliness are common during treatment and the possibility of relapse after treatment is over add weight to those feelings. Providing privacy and maintaining dignity for children whatever their age is just as important as it is for adult patients.

NUTRITION

Sufficient intake of food to grow and thrive is necessary for all living beings. Children especially have nutritional needs that must be met for normal growth and development. All illness and especially chronic illness such as cancer militate against this, so early intervention and prevention are necessary.

On admission a full dietary assessment including likes, dislikes, normal patterns of eating, language used for foods and implements used at home should be recorded in the care plan and followed closely. Baseline weights and heights are taken and recorded on a centile chart as well as graphed for later comparison. Regular weight checks and the use of percentile charts are needed both to monitor changes and to ensure that drug doses are calculated accurately. Children of all age groups will frequently improve their nutritional intake if given a choice and if involved in filling in their nutritional chart.

A poor nutritional status may be caused by the disease itself; a tumour may cause a protein-losing enteropathy, catecholamine release from neuroblastoma reduces appetite, a tumour mass can make eating uncomfortable, and electrolyte imbalance may reduce or interfere with food tolerance.

Malabsorption may occur as a result of the disease or as a side-effect of treatment. Nearly all cytotoxic chemotherapy induces nausea and vomiting and some may cause diarrhoea or constipation. High-dose chemotherapy can damage the gastro-intestinal lining so that malabsorption of nutrients follows. Chemotherapy affects the mucous membranes of the mouth leading to mucositis and an associated unwillingness to eat. Radiotherapy depending on the irradiated area will have similar effects on the mouth and gastrointestinal tract while some surgery will necessitate periods without oral intake at all.

Prevention of weight loss should be the aim from the day of diagnosis. All families have different eating patterns, many children are fussy eaters, hospital catering is not always to the liking of the children, and the temptation to allow a sick child to eat whatever he fancies is great. Care planning needs to involve our health education role with easily understood help and advice being offered to families whose own eating habits may not be ideal. Some well children are poor eaters, most thrive despite this and, although encouraging a normal diet is important, it should be done in as relaxed manner as possible. Mealtimes should not be allowed to become a battleground and especially conflict between the parents and child should be avoided. Such antagonism can harm their crucial relationship and if eating (or lack of it) becomes an obsession, serious family disruption may follow.

The maintenance of mealtimes is important. The social act of eating in the dining room with other children should be the norm whenever possible, especially for younger children who may be given encouragement by peer support rather than being cajoled by an anxious mother or nurse.

Appropriate and nutritious food is important; however, sweets or chocolate as a reward after meals can boost the child's morale as well as having calorific value. Crisps seem to be popular, even for children with apparently sore mouths, and are a good source of calories.

The provision of cooking facilities for parents on the ward helps as the likelihood of children eating food seen to be prepared by their own mother is greater. Parents' ability to provide food outside hospital mealtimes for children with decreased appetites as a result of treatments known to cause nausea and vomiting such as cytotoxic drugs is a great advantage.

The only caution with parents providing food on the ward is in its microbiological safety, because cancer treatments affect the child's vulnerability to infection. Strict hygiene must be observed and food stored safely. A discreet educational programme for families at the outset of their stay should be initiated, emphasising hand-washing and always cooking food thoroughly. Re-heated or saved food needs special attention. It must be cooked through and not allowed to partly thaw and then be refrozen.

Some patients, usually those that are seriously immuno-suppressed, either because of chemotherapy or during bone marrow transplantation, may require very stringent dietary restrictions involving specially prepared and cooked food, as well as restrictions on fresh foods, such as salads and fruit. Guidelines vary from institution to institution but optimal safety with few restrictions should be the aim. It is, however, very important to develop reasonable guidelines and practice with clear written instruction for everyone in the unit.

Children from families with different cultural beliefs and from different ethnic backgrounds present a particular challenge. Hospital food is often unpalatable to them, even if it is Kosher or Halal. Particular care and sensitivity in providing the child with a suitable diet is important. Relatives will frequently bring in food from home for the child and the parent.

Regular weight checks are needed throughout treatment. Sudden gains and losses must be explained. A course of oral steroids may increase both appetite and weight rapidly but it is usually a temporary gain.

If oral nutrition fails to improve the child's nutritional status and weight gain, other routes should be considered. Oral caloric content of food can be increased by using high-calorie and high-energy supplements; most of these are well tolerated by children if presented carefully.

Nasogastric feed supplements at night are a useful additional source of calories and can take the pressure and unhappiness out of trying to eat more than they want during the day. The passing of a nasogastric tube is unpleasant but once in situ is usually well tolerated and can remain there for some time. High-calorie feeds such as *Ensure* provide high calorific values but need to be built up gradually for tolerance. Initially, diarrhoea or vomiting may occur if introduced too quickly. A severely malnourished child can often be sent home on enteral feeding. A return to home is often the key to improving a child's nutritional intake. The child feeling happier at home will often return to eating and drinking normally!

If the enteral route is unsuitable it may be necessary to commence intravenous feeding. This is usually considered to be a last resort and should be short-term; as soon as the body recovers from the cancer treatment enteral feeding can recommence.

Intravenous feeding can either be through a peripheral venous line or a central venous catheter (Figure 3.1). Peripheral

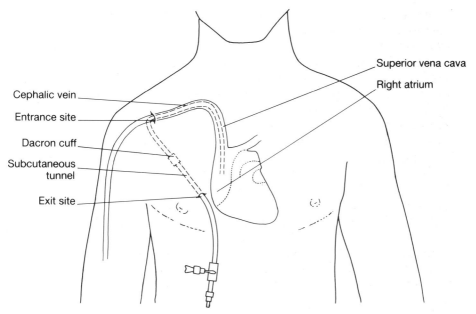

Figure 3.1   Diagram of the anatomical relationship in the placement of a tunnelled central venous catheter

feeding is not as successful as the strength of solution has to be limited due to potential venous damage. Any extravasation of fluid can be dangerous because of the electrolytes added to the solution and leakages may cause burning, tissue necrosis and lasting damage requiring subsequent skin grafting. Feeding through a central venous catheter, such as a Hickman line, is much more successful as good calorie intake is easier to achieve.

Problems may occur when a high calorie intake is suddenly introduced to a malnourished body. The strength of intravenous feed must be increased gradually, electrolytes checked daily and the solution adjusted accordingly. Body weight is checked and recorded daily and blood sugar checked every six hours to begin with. A daily urinalysis looking especially for sugar will also warn of sugar overload. All these parameters must be clearly outlined at the beginning of total parenteral nutrition and regularly recorded while therapy continues.

BONE MARROW SUPPRESSION

Radiotherapy and chemotherapy may induce bone marrow suppression where there is underproduction of red and white blood cells and platelets. This causes anaemia, a bleeding tendency and poor resistance to infection if not regulated. Anaemia is usually defined as a haemoglobin below 8 g/dl and may be caused by the disease or the treatment. Careful nursing of the child can reduce the impact of anaemia by conserving energy and reducing fatigue. Regular blood checks should be undertaken and haemoglobin levels corrected with packed cell transfusion before the child becomes too lethargic and tired. Quiet periods and restful games as well as minimising activities can help to conserve energy. Parents need to understand the affects of anaemia and are often able to gauge their own child's haemoglobin level by his activity level.

Thrombocytopenia, a reduction in the platelet content of the blood (normal range 150–450 × 10^9/l), is frequently a problem while cancer treatment is being given. Platelet transfusions are now commonly given to avoid bleeding problems. A platelet count of below 50 × 10^9/l can be troublesome to some patients with signs of bleeding apparent; many may have a count as low as 20 × 10^9/l before routine platelet transfusion is required.

If bleeding does occur it is likely to be in the form of epistaxis, petechiae, bruising or bleeding gums. A careful nursing assessment of the patient each day should reveal any new problems and parents can be taught to assess their child at bath time. Boisterous games or activities likely to cause trauma and bleeding are not encouraged but can be difficult to suppress!

Intramuscular injections are avoided where possible. If they have to be given, the platelet count must be checked first and the puncture site carefully observed.

More serious gastrointestinal bleeding may occur. For this reason aspirin products are not used, paracetamol being given for pain relief or reduction of fever.

Both red cell and platelet transfusions are now commonplace for children with cancer, but are not without hazard. Despite highly sophisticated cross-matching, problems do occur and antibodies are formed making subsequent transfusions more difficult. Baseline observations of temperature, pulse and respirations should precede transfusion and be followed by routine observation throughout. Side-effects include nausea, vomiting, headache, rigors and rashes but these usually respond to intravenous antihistamine and steroid therapy. Subsequent transfusions should be preceded by prophylactic medications.

INFECTION

All rapidly dividing cells in the bone marrow are affected by chemotherapy and radiotherapy. Thrombocytopenia and anaemia are relatively easily controlled with blood and platelet transfusion. The effect on the white cells, particularly neutrophils, renders the patient highly susceptible to infection, particularly when the absolute neutrophil count falls below $0.5 \times 10^9/l$. At this level the patient is at risk from his environment and from his own gut flora.

Signs of infection may be masked as there are no white cells to form pus or inflammation around a wound. Minor infections that would not affect a healthy patient may produce a systemic septicaemia in the immunosuppressed child causing high morbidity or mortality. As treatments for the less responsive cancers become more intensive, risks from infection increase. The longer the child is neutropenic the greater the risk. Much can be done by the nursing staff to make sure the child is protected. It is important to teach the family where the potential hazards lie and so avoid taking risks. It is policy on some units to nurse severely neutropenic patients in isolation, while other centres endeavour to provide a 'clean' environment for all patients by using air filtration. Isolation is hard on the child but may be necessary, particularly during bone marrow transplantation.

Once an infective agent affects a neutropenic child the course can be rapidly fatal so prevention and early detection are nursing priorities. Daily evaluation of the patient and diligence in maintaining a microbiologically safe environment help. A four-hourly observation of the temperature is a good indicator and parents will soon learn to monitor and report any rises themselves. Any rise in temperature is taken seriously; the patient has specimens of blood, urine, stool, throat and nose swabs taken for culture. If a Hickman catheter is in situ both central and peripheral blood cultures must be taken in case the line is infected. Any headache or neck stiffness should be investigated by lumbar puncture.

Routine weekly or twice-weekly specimen screening will give guidelines should infection subsequently occur. Basic hygiene must be scrupulous with careful handwashing being most important. Regular washing, bathing, careful cleaning of the mouth after eating and the perineum after micturition and defaecation will lessen the risk of infection. Any skin lesions should be carefully cleaned and reported. Keeping the ward clean and uncluttered should be encouraged and flowers or plants in the ward area removed as they may carry bacteria, and the water may carry *Pseudomonas*. As already discussed, food should be safely prepared and carefully supervised. There should be careful avoidance of contact with communicable diseases such as measles and chicken-pox.

Despite very careful care, febrile illnesses during periods of neutropenia are common. Early intervention with broad spectrum intravenous antibiotics is routine and often highly effective, though it is important that blood cultures are taken before drugs are given. As a result of antibiotic therapy *Candida* may be present so routine prophylactic antifungal treatment is given orally. It must be given regularly and kept in the mouth for as long as possible for maximum effect.

While febrile the child will often be miserable. Regular antipyretics such as paracetamol will help. Cool cotton clothing and good fluid intake also help. Children with cancer are at risk from infection as long as the white blood count remains low. Some therapies render the white blood count low for some time necessitating several courses of antibiotics or several antibiotics, antiviral and antifungal agents in combination. A child on many different drugs all given intravenously presents the oncology nurse with new problems. She must safely administer the drugs to the child at the prescribed intervals while ensuring they do not react with each other and the child does not become overloaded with fluid.

Intravenous therapy in the child with cancer is often complex. One catheter may be used for antibiotic, antiviral/antifungal agents, blood and platelet supportive therapy, antihistamine and steroid therapy, cytotoxic drugs and parenteral nutrition all in one day. This provides a challenge to the nursing staff administering care. Good venous access is essential and tunnelled central venous catheters have improved the quality of life for these children enormously, though they are in themselves a possible route for infection. All central venous catheters must be handled using an aseptic technique. Between courses of treatment they are flushed with a heparin saline solution and sealed. The frequency of heparinisation of central lines varies and local policies exist. Most parents are taught to do this initially in hospital and continue at home without difficulty. It is sometimes possible in the less seriously ill child to have a course of intravenous antibiotics given at home by the parents.

Infection is still a problem when the child goes home. Although the white cell count will have recovered, the immunity will still be impaired leaving the child vulnerable to viral infections and especially common childhood illnesses such as measles and chicken-pox. Although normal activity, school and play are encouraged, any contact with measles and chicken-pox should be notified and immunoglobulins given. There is still no drug available against measles in the inmunosuppressed and although rare, some children with cancer die from it. Chicken-pox is now treatable with acyclovir but should still be avoided.

SYMPTOM RELIEF

Nausea

A common, unpleasant and difficult-to-treat side-effect of cancer therapy is nausea and vomiting. Anti-emetics do work for some patients. Children on the whole cope well with this distressing side-effect and recover quickly from it. Some prefer not to take anti-emetics at all as they do not like the soporific effect they have. Some develop an intolerance to the drugs themselves and so cannot take them. In general, children receiving repeated courses of treatment usually know what they want to take. Some seem not to mind the vomiting and accept it. Commonly used drugs include metoclopramide (Maxolon) and prochlorperazine (Stemetil). A cannabis derivative, nabilone, given orally prophylactically is now being used with some success.

Mouth Care

Several cytotoxic drugs cause another distressing side-effect, mucositis. In addition, a neutropenic patient may well have oral *Candida* or even herpetic lesions, all adding to his misery. Scrupulous hygiene and good prophylactic mouth care is the best way round this difficult problem and is one of the first facets of care most parents learn. Gentle, regular toothbrushing with a soft brush is to be encouraged in older children with mouthwashes using a suitable agent between times. The child under eight years will need help with toothbrushing to ensure it is properly carried out.

Regular inspections of the mouth should take place and care is adjusted accordingly. The services of a dentist are encouraged. Many regional centres have a dentist as part of their team to help and advise on good dental care. Regular check-ups should take place throughout cancer treatment and any dental treatment needed done in hospital.

SUMMARY

The initial suspicion of childhood cancer and the subsequent bewildering procedures around the diagnostic period are extremely fraught for the child and his family. To be admitted to the strange environment of a busy hospital, surrounded by other families in a similar situation and then having to take in so much new information is daunting.

It is important for paediatric oncology nurses to support, educate and be available to discuss issues with all these families in a way that each will understand. Parents often remark that they would never have dreamt they could be so actively involved in medical and nursing care of their own child before treatment, but most are anxious to be involved and keen to do whatever they can. By role modelling and offering consistent sound advice, we are able to help them to achieve this.

Further Reading

Arnfield A (1985) Children's tumours. In: *Nursing the Patient with Cancer* Tschudin V (ed.). New York: Prentice Hall.

Hockenberry M and Coody D (1986) *Paediatric Haematology and Oncology – Perspectives in Care*. St Louis: C V Mosby.

Oakhill A (1988) *The Supportive Care of the Child with Cancer*, 2nd edn. Berlin: Springer-Verlag.

Voûte P A, Barratt A, Bloom H V G, Lemerle V and Neidhart M K (eds.) (1986) *Cancer in Children, Clinical Management*, 2 edn. Berlin: Springer-Verlag.

4

Investigations, Staging and Diagnosis – Implications for Nurses

Until twenty years ago there was little purpose in subjecting children to numerous unpleasant tests to confirm the diagnosis of cancer as there was virtually no treatment to offer, but today this is no longer the case. Confirming the diagnosis and measuring the amount and spread of the disease play a very important part in the planning of treatment and assessing the overall prognosis.

Cancer is no longer viewed as a life-threatening disease but as a chronic illness. The increase in the cure and survival rates, even in children with metastatic disease, has resulted in the need for more accurate methods of diagnosing and staging paediatric tumours:

- The diagnosis of a malignant disease in a child is an emergency – not necessarily a medical emergency but an emotional one. To some parents in this situation, a paediatric illness with a worse prognosis may seem preferable to that of cancer. To others, the suspicion and waiting is worse, the confirmation comes almost, as a relief. (Barbor, 1983).

When cancer is first suspected the child and his family may be referred to a specialist centre. For this reason even if the general practitioner or paediatrician has not voiced his suspicions, the parents and child may be anxious about being referred to a special hospital or ward. If the parents are not prepared or have not had time to come to terms with the fact that their child may have cancer, they may find the confrontation with other children who have a malignant disease difficult. Sharing a ward with children undergoing treatment and observing some of the obvious side-effects, e.g. alopecia, nausea and vomiting, may be too much for the child and his parents to cope with.

However, if the parents have been transferred from a unit where their child was the only one with a suspected malignancy, they may well be relieved to be in an area where they are no longer being treated as 'abnormal'. The child and his parents may well have felt isolated by being the only one with cancer. Other parents find difficulty in knowing what to say and often prefer to say nothing for fear of upsetting other members of the family.

Preparation may facilitate an easier or more comfortable admission for all the family. A general practitioner may only see one case of childhood cancer during his career and it is therefore unrealistic to expect him to know about the oncology unit to which he refers the child and his family. However, this should not prevent him enquiring when the occasion arises. Booklets or leaflets giving basic information about the facilities available in a specialist unit, the telephone numbers and any other relevant information can be of use and value for general practitioners and referring hospitals.

Nurses working in the field of paediatric oncology need to be aware of and prepared for the variety of reactions and emotions from the child and his family on their first admission. The most important thing that we as nurses can give at this stage is reassurance, not a blanket statement that everything will be all right, or that it is not cancer, but that everything that needs to be done to reach a diagnosis will be done as quickly and efficiently as possible. Also that the family will be involved and kept up to date with any information about their child and his disease. Parents will need reassurance that feelings of anger, fear, shock, disbelief, grief and guilt are not unusual and need to be expressed.

Although the parents may find it difficult socially and emotionally to be away from home, the patient will ultimately benefit. Paediatric oncology units have the facilities to carry out all or most of the investigations within the one hospital. Such units have experienced staff to plan procedures with the minimum of stress to the child and have access to experts who will interpret the results of the investigations.

Paediatric oncology nurses require knowledge based on reasons for the variety of diagnostic tests and investigations that need to be carried out to confirm the diagnosis of the tumour or leukaemia. If we do not possess this basic knowledge, including an understanding of why and how the tests are performed, what, if any, preparation is needed, or how long the procedure lasts, we cannot assist with the preparation of the child and his family to undergo efficient diagnostic work-up.

The introduction of a primary nurse at this stage can be of tremendous help to the child and his family. A primary nurse can support the child and family by providing a physical and psychological environment that facilitates the establishment of a good relationship. She can encourage the parents to participate in the care of their child and establish the extent that they feel able to do so. This in turn helps the child settle in and helps us to find out more about him. The parents possess a wealth of information about their child, the primary nurse possesses the knowledge regarding the investigation and treatment of the suspected disease; by working together they can prepare the child for the various tests he will undergo. There may not be enough time to establish trusting relationships with the patient before the investigations begin, but by encouraging the parents to work alongside the staff, preparation and education can take place simultaneously. Parents provide the information on the type of preparation their child will need, whether he requires prior knowledge and time to act things out, time to ask questions, the opportunity to view instruments or equipment, to observe someone else undergoing the procedure, or whether he needs to be told immediately prior to the procedure.

Kubler Ross (1970) said in relation to dying that 'everyone has a right to know that they are dying but not everyone needs to know'. I would suggest that this applies to children undergoing unpleasant, uncomfortable or painful procedures. If we have not had the time or opportunity to build up a relationship at this stage with the patient, the parents are of invaluable help in deciding or assisting in the decision of what the child needs to know and when he needs to know it, to enable him to cope.

Whenever possible, the primary nurse should attend the interviews that the doctors have with the parents and child. Knowing the information and terminology that has been given to the parents will enable the primary nurse to clarify and explain anything that the parents did not understand. It is not unusual for parents not to hear or understand the rest of the conversation once the name of the tumour or the word 'cancer' has been used.

It was stated previously that there is a need for the investigations to be planned efficiently with the minimum amount of physical and psychological trauma to the patient. Fotchman et al (1982) agrees that it cannot be stressed enough that in order for the child to accept not only the investigations but the treatment and survive emotionally, he must be prepared psychologically. Children may be 'brave' for one procedure, but children with leukaemia, for example, face numerous invasive procedures, e.g. bone marrow aspirates, and therefore if they are to cooperate and comply with such procedures and the following treatment, it is at this stage that an acceptable way must be found to assist the child through each procedure.

There are several methods that can be of value to children facing such procedures.

General Anaesthesia

General anaesthesia permits multiple invasive or painful procedures to be performed without causing discomfort to the child. They can usually be carried out in most departments, for example, the scanning or X-ray department. Analgesia can be administered before the child is fully awake, thereby preventing or alleviating immediate discomfort from multiple procedures. Preoperative fasting may cause the child to become anxious; it is not uncommon for children who have been refusing oral fluids prior to a preoperative fast to start demanding fluids on the commencement of the fast. Children may have experienced previous general anaesthesia and may have anxieties or fears about it. They should be encouraged to talk in order to allay fears and, if possible, prevent a similar occurrence happening again. Some children find the smell of the anaesthetic mask is unpleasant or have a fear of the mask being placed over their nose and mouth. Parents again are of invaluable help in reassuring and comforting their child in the anaesthetic room. Paediatric anaesthetists need all their skills in gaining the child's cooperation and a flexible approach is much appreciated by the child, parents and nurses. The use of an aromatic oil applied to the face mask and allowing the child to be cuddled by a parent until he or she is drowsy are conducive to a less traumatic anaesthetic induction. The use of intravenous anaesthetic drugs should be offered to a child if necessary. It is important to carry out pre-anaesthetic investigations of the child's basic blood count if bone marrow disease is suspected. A low haemoglobin may be an indication to delay the procedure until corrective measures are carried out.

Ketamine is a short-acting anaesthetic that can be administered intravenously. Children require a preoperative fast and should not be woken suddenly or be subjected to loud noises as they are waking up as they can experience nightmares or hallucinations.

Local Anaesthesia

Local anaesthesia is usually administered by an injection. It therefore requires a cooperative child who can 'cope' with an injection and be able to remain in the position they are placed in for the procedure. If a local anaesthetic is being used because the child's clinical condition contraindicates general anaesthesia, i.e. a large mediastinal mass or a very low haemoglobin, a sedative may be required to facilitate cooperation and prevent an increase in anxiety. Topical anaesthetic creams or sprays, such as Emla cream, may also be of value. Emla cream contains lignocaine and prilocaine. These can be applied to skin around the area where the needle will be introduced to induce local anaesthesia. Topical anaesthetic creams are valuable when siting cannulae or performing other procedures that require children to receive an injection or needle puncture. Entonox (CO_2 + NO) can be used for older children who are able to hold the mask and self-administer the gas. It can be used as a form of diversional therapy giving the child something else to concentrate on.

Sedation is required by children who are anxious about forthcoming procedures. Single agents are not usually effective to allow uncomfortable procedures being performed without the patient waking up. A combination of sedatives and analgesics have been found to be more effective.

One such cocktail is trimeprazine, droperidol and methadone. This medication is administered orally a minimum of 1.5 hours prior to the planned procedure. This sedation usually facilitates children being moved from one position to another or even between departments. If painful procedures are carried out the child will wake but is usually easily placated and will return to sleep on completion of the procedure. The disadvantage of using this type of sedation is the length of time it may take the child to wake fully. It is not advisable, therefore, for long-term daily use because of the time 'lost' each day. Although fasting is not a requirement, the child will sleep through at least one meal and may experience altered nocturnal sleeping patterns having slept for 4–5 hours during the day. This medication is useful when placing cannulae as it allows time for the veins to be examined without creating anxiety in the child. If such procedures can be planned for late afternoon or evening, the child will not miss out on too much social activity.

Relaxation has been found to be valuable to older children. Teaching the parents the method of relaxation and encouraging them to participate in the exercises may also benefit them as well as their child. If trusting relationships have not yet been fully established the patient may not have the confidence in being able to use it fully.

It is important to remember that all children are individuals. Their experiences in life, and in hospital particularly, are individual and so their needs are individual too. There should be no rules or regulations governing the age of children 'allowed' to have a general anaesthesia or sedation for any procedures. Flexibility is important. Should a child decide upon a certain method to cope with his investigations, he should not be expected to continue with that method if it is found to be unsuitable for subsequent procedures.

INVESTIGATION AND STAGING

Multiple investigations may be required to establish an accurate diagnosis. Staging procedures are carried out to evaluate the spread of the disease. There are different staging or classification systems. One widely used system is the 'TNM' system. This system involves evaluation in three groups:

1 Tumour – the size of the primary
2 Node – the involvement of the regional lymph nodes
3 Metastasis – the involvement of distant organs

Numerical sub-headings are then used to denote the stage or extent of involvement. A small tumour with no nodal involvement and no evidence of distant metastasis would be reported as T1NOMO.

TNM patterns can also be grouped into stages:

- Stage I – local disease only
- Stage II – regional disease
- Stage III – metastatic disease.

The importance of staging varies with different tumours but is important for determining the need for local or systemic treatment. In leukaemia it does little to determine the overall prognosis. In Hodgkin's disease, however, staging is relative not only to the prognosis, but also to the type and extent of treatment.

RADIOLOGICAL INVESTIGATIONS

Conventional radiography has an important role to play in aiding the diagnosis and staging of childhood cancers.

Plain X-rays may display the characteristics and fine detail of specific tumours, e.g. bone tumours, or may be able to identify areas of calcification in a mass, e.g. neuroblastoma. X-rays are not invasive to children – they do not 'hurt' but they do require the child's cooperation either to remain still, to control breathing or to allow the X-ray machine or film near their body.

X-ray departments working with children usually develop or design ideas that are conducive to putting a child at ease and gaining his trust and cooperation: allowing the children to play with some of the switches, having pictures and mobiles suitably placed, and allowing the parents to be in view or within hearing help. Plain X-rays do not require any physical preparation. The psychological preparation will depend on age and any previous experience the child may have had. Explanations and reassurance from the parents, radiographer and nurse are vital.

LYMPHOGRAPHY

Until recently, lymphography was the only way to identify involved lymph nodes. The procedure is painful due to the administration of a contrast via the lymphatic vessels. These are isolated in the interdigital space in the patient's foot via a small cut-down procedure. Once the contrast is administered the patient is required to lie still until all the lymph nodes have been identified on X-ray. Sutures following the cut-down procedures will restrict the shoes that the child can wear. If the patient is having this test as an outpatient, the parents will need advice about suitable footwear. Follow-up X-rays are required 24–48 hours later. The contrast administered is blue and will result in a change in the child's complexion. His urine will also be coloured. Both will fade and disappear as the contrast is excreted but the child and family need pre-warning.

Using this information the nurse needs to discuss with the parents the best way to prepare the patient. A general anaesthetic or sedation may be used. Diversional therapy will be required if the patient chooses to stay awake. Tape recorders with favourite stories or songs are useful.

Lymphograms are primarily required in the staging of children with Hodgkin's disease.

COMPUTERISED AXIAL TOMOGRAPHY SCANNING (CAT OR CT)

CT scanning was introduced into clinical practice in 1973. CT scans give a more accurate picture of the size of the tumour and the relationship to the surrounding organs and structures.

CT scans may be taken of the whole body or specific parts, e.g. pelvis, abdomen, chest, etc. Contrast medium may be given orally or intravenously to specify the vessels or organ, and to enhance normal tissue parenchyma.

CT scans are not painful. The procedure may require the child to fast – usually for two hours prior to the scan if oral contrast is to be administered. Encouraging children to drink the contrast requires patience and help from the parents.

The scan requires that children remain still and, if the lungs are to be scanned, breathing also has to be controlled. Young children who are frightened of the machine, or unable to comply with the restrictions of movement and breath control, may require sedation or general anaesthesia (Figure 4.1). The use of general anaesthesia means that oral contrast cannot be given and may result in a less easily definable scan. Sedation does not facilitate control of breathing and therefore cannot be used for chest scans. Time spent in preparing the child to be able to cope and cooperate may avoid the use of an anaesthetic or sedation and result in a more easily definable scan.

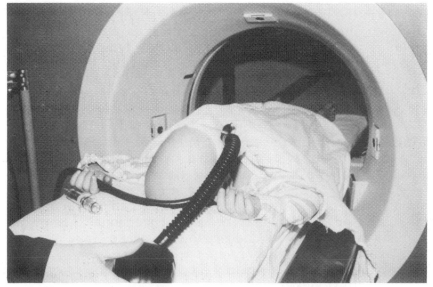

Figure 4.1   A small child has a general anaesthetic for a CAT scan

DIAGNOSTIC ULTRASOUND

Ultrasound procedures are non-invasive and non-threatening. A feeling of pressure or discomfort may be experienced if there is local swelling or distention at the tumour site.

There is no physical preparation other than a full bladder for pelvic scans. Mothers who have experienced ultrasound scans during pregnancy will be able to reassure their child and allay or prevent anxiety. The staff in the department can help by providing a friendly relaxed atmosphere. Encouraging the parents to stay, explaining the procedure step by step and allowing diversional therapy, e.g. story tapes, all help.

Sedation may be required for children who are unable to lie still.

NUCLEAR MEDICINE SCANS

These are scans using gamma cameras and radiopharmaceuticals or isotopes. The isotopes are administered intravenously and the scan is performed at a specified time. The timing is dependent upon the length of time the isotope takes to concentrate in the specific organ.

There is no physical preparation but an empty bladder is required for a pelvic scan.

Providing venous access is available, the scans (Figure 4.2) are non-threatening and painless. It does require the patient to lie still and therefore sedation may be required. If venous access is not available the sedative cocktail mentioned earlier is of particular value. It facilitates the adminstration of the isotope without causing undue stress or trauma to the child and he then remains sedated for the scan.

MIBG (Meta-iodobenzylguanidine)

This is a scan using radioactive iodine. It is used specifically to detect neuroblastoma, a malignant disease of the sympathetic nervous system, and phaeochromocytoma, a catecholamine producing tumour (usually benign) of the sympathetic-adrenal system. The preparation is as for other radioactive isotope scans. The psychological preparation for all these scans requires explanation and reassurance from the parents and the nurse. Visits to the scanning room, observing the equipment and watching another child undergoing a scan may be of value.

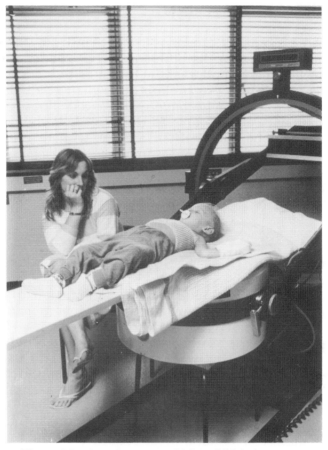

Figure 4.2   A mother stays with her child during a scan

HAEMATOLOGICAL INVESTIGATIONS

Blood tests become a regular occurrence for most children with cancer. This does not mean, however, that we can assume that children will be able to cope because they have experienced them before. On the contrary, some children's anxieties increase at the thought of having more or repeated blood tests.

Venous access needs to be established with the least amount of trauma to the child. The general condition of the patient will indicate whether time is available to find a method that is acceptable. Sedation as previously mentioned is extremely useful, as it allows time to identify the most suitable vein and facilitates other investigations such as a general physical examination which a younger child may not have accepted previously.

Establishing which is the dominant hand and choosing, if possible, a vein on the other limb makes it easier for the child to participate in everyday activities.

The placement of a central venous line such as a Hickman, Broviac or Portacath should be seriously considered at this stage. If the child is to undergo investigations that require a general anaesthetic and the disease suspected requires treatment with repeated chemotherapy agents, it is advantageous to place a central venous line at this time, preventing a repeated anaesthetic and delay in commencing treatment.

Preparation of a child for this procedure may include demonstrating the advantages of the line using another child with an existing line, e.g. taking blood samples and giving 'injections'. Children who have been subjected to multiple blood tests do not usually need much persuasion to have a central line – some even request it. Attention can be drawn to the fact that there are no restrictions on their arms when infusions are in progress so mobilisation and play are easier.

The play therapist has an important role in providing and encouraging play with dolls or teddy bears that have lines attached to them and can help children act out their fears or anxieties. Children frequently name their lines, e.g. wiggly or worm, and time spent choosing a special name will help as diversional therapy and acceptance.

Baseline blood values are required to assess the clinical condition of the patient and to aid diagnosis. Blood products and electrolyte replacement infusions may be required before the patient's condition is stable enough to undergo further investigations, for example, a child with thrombocytopenia will require a platelet transfusion prior to an invasive procedure such as a lumbar puncture.

Some tumours produce marker substances either biochemical or protein that can be measured or assessed in the blood or urine. Such markers can aid diagnosis, i.e. when found to be in excess of normal limits, and can then be used to monitor the response to treatment. Examples of markers are alpha-fetoprotein (AFP) measured in the blood, elevated levels of which indicate a yolk sac tumour. Vanillyelmandelic acid (VMA) is a biochemical marker measured in the urine. An elevated level is found in children with neuroblastoma.

Bone marrow aspiration and biopsy are performed to verify evidence of disease in the bone marrow as in leukaemia or malignant diseases that may have metastasised to the marrow, for example, neuroblastoma. Bone marrow aspiration is a painful and uncomfortable procedure. Some children may require only one bone marrow investigation to establish a diagnosis. Children with leukaemia will have repeated investigations. Once again, it is important to establish a method that will enable the child to cope with the procedure. Local anaesthesia helps but the procedure is still uncomfortable, both from the position the child is required to adopt and the amount of pressure that is required to obtain the specimen. The suction applied via the syringe is also painful. For younger or anxious children facing multiple investigations, a general anaesthetic is preferable. The child may experience pain or tenderness at the site of the bone marrow test especially if a biopsy is also taken and adequate regular analgesia may be required. The psychological assessment and preparation for this procedure especially for the child with leukaemia is important.

Other haematological investigations may be requested to aid in the general assessment of the child's condition and to enable corrective measures to be taken prior to the commencement of treatment. Providing that adequate venous access has been established the numerous requests for blood samples should not prove to be too traumatic for the child.

SURGICAL PROCEDURES/BIOPSIES

Biopsies, needle aspirations and lumbar punctures are all invasive, painful procedures. In addition to the pain from the procedure the child may be required to lie in an uncomfortable position. Lumbar punctures come in this category. They require the child's complete cooperation – movement at a critical moment can result in unnecessary trauma or damage. It may be acceptable to hold a young baby in the position for a lumbar puncture but it is both difficult and may be damaging psychologically to hold a child against his will. Sedation or general anaesthesia again provides a means to help children through this and other surgical procedures.

CONCLUSION

Fotchman and Foley (1982) and Culling (1988) state that the investigations carried out to establish the diagnosis of cancer must be well planned to prevent children experiencing physical or psychological harm. When general anaesthesia or sedation are required as many as necessary procedures as possible should be carried out during the time the child is asleep. This will prevent the child having repeated anaesthetics or sedatives. Close liaison and cooperation between many departments is necessary to set a convenient time and place to carry out such procedures.

The nurse's role in preparing the child and educating the parents is very important. Kratz et al (1980) found that increased anxiety especially in young children was related to medical procedures. Kratz et al (1980) also commented that there was insufficient evidence to suggest that any one single method of preparation has better results. Treating each child as an individual – assessing his needs with his parents and planning individual realistic goals – establishes a good basis for gaining the child's trust and cooperation.

Information booklets, leaflets and photograph albums of children undergoing various procedures are also very useful. Ward mascots displayed as badges or pictures in other departments can be helpful when the child is meeting new people away from the ward environment.

It has already been stated that the parents need a tremendous amount of support and education during the investigation period. Their education is not just about the child's illness and treatment but how to cope with it and how to help their child and the rest of the family cope.

Parents need to be kept up to date. Results and implications of the results should be explained to them. As soon as the diagnosis is reached the parents need to be informed. The child's primary nurse should also attend this interview between parents and the doctor. Once the parents have heard the diagnosis and had time and the opportunity to ask questions preparation for telling the patient and rest of the family must start.

According to Kratz et al (1980), the ability of a child and his family to survive emotionally following the diagnosis of cancer is related to the psychological care and support that they receive during the diagnostic phase and early part of their treatment. The role of the paediatric oncology nurse is to provide an environment that is conducive to the physical and emotional well-being of the child and his family. To do this she must possess sound knowledge in order to educate, prepare and forward plan the care of the child and his family.

References

Barbor P (1983) Emotional aspects of malignant disease in children. *Maternal and Child Health.* 320–327.

Culling J A (1988) The psychological problems of families of children with cancer. In: *The Supportive Care of the Child with Cancer*, Oakhill A. London: Wright.

Fotchman D and Foley G (1982) *Nursing Care of the Child with Cancer.* Boston: Little, Brown.

Fotchman D, Ferguson J, Ford N and Pryor A (1982) The treatment of cancer in children. In: *Nursing Care of the Child with Cancer*, chapter 5. Boston: Little, Brown.

Koocher G P and O'Malley J E (1981) *The Damocles Syndrome.* New York: McGraw-Hill.

Kratz E R, Kellerman J and Seigel S (1980) Behavioural distress in children undergoing medical procedures; development considerations. *Journal of Consultant Clinical Psychology*, **49**(3): 470–1.

Kubler-Ross E (1970) *On Death and Dying.* London: Tavistock.

5
The Child Receiving Chemotherapy

The advent of combination chemotherapy in the 1970s has vastly improved the outlook for children with cancer. Before that time, when single-agent chemotherapy was used, childhood cancer was an acute terminal illness; today it is a chronic illness with a 60–70 per cent survival rate.

HOW CYTOTOXIC DRUGS ACT

A cancer, whether a solid tumour or leukaemia, is defined as an abnormal proliferation of rapidly dividing cells, in which the number of cells produced.exceeds the number of cells lost. The body's control mechanism for cell division fails.

Cytotoxic (cell-killing) drugs act by interfering with cell division and growth to arrest the formation of new cancer cells. They are the only therapeutic option for leukaemias and lymphomas where disease is disseminated. They are also used either to shrink a tumour before surgery or to 'mop up' tumour cells following surgery or radiotherapy. In some cases, cells may break away from the original tumour to form distant metastases; again chemotherapy is the treatment of choice.

CELL-CYCLE KINETICS

Before cell division or mitosis can occur, the deoxyribonucleic acid (DNA) contained in the nucleus of the cell must be doubled. DNA is synthesised from metabolites within the cell during a fairly short time interval, and this is preceded and followed by resting phases in the cell cycle (Figure 5.1). Cells that are not actively dividing but have the capacity to proliferate are said to be in the Go phase. The principle behind giving combinations of cytotoxic drugs is that they have differing modes of action on cell division and growth – some act at certain phases of the cell cycle (cell cycle-specific), while others

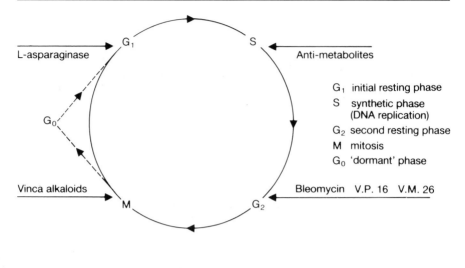

L-asparaginase

Anti-metabolites

G_1　initial resting phase
S　synthetic phase
　　(DNA replication)
G_2　second resting phase
M　mitosis
G_0　'dormant' phase

Vinca alkaloids

Bleomycin　V.P. 16　V.M. 26

Cell cycle-non-specific drugs
Alkylating agents
Antimitotic antibiotics

Figure 5.1　The cell cycle, with main sites of action of common cell cycle-specific cytotoxic drugs

are non-specific (cell cycle-non-specific) and act by interfering with the structure of DNA in various ways (see Figure 5.1). Thus, in theory, all phases of the cell cycle are affected, and it is clear that the timing of giving combination chemotherapy is critical.

The timing of giving courses of drugs is also critical; toxicity to normal tissues must be carefully balanced against toxicity to cancer cells. Following drug therapy both tumour cells and rapidly dividing normal cells are damaged but tumour cell recovery is slower than that of normal cells. The principle behind giving 'pulsed' chemotherapy relies on this theory and exploits the poor recovery of tumour cells (Figure 5.2). If the interval between courses is too short, progressive toxicity to normal cells occurs; if the interval is too long tumour cells will recover and treatment will be ineffective. Since the bone marrow is the most sensitive normal tissue, recovery of normal cells is monitored by blood counts which reflect bone marrow activity. Treatment is given when the neutrophil count is 1.0×10^9/l and above and the platelet count is greater than 100×10^9/l.

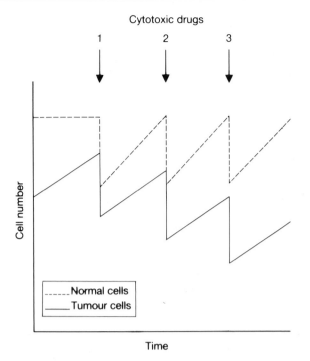

Figure 5.2   Pulsed chemotherapy

DRUG RESISTANCE

It is possible for tumours to become resistant to cytotoxic drugs, where neutralising antibodies are directed against the drug. Giving combination chemotherapy in high doses should pre-empt this problem. Lack of response may simply be due to failure of the drug to reach the tumour; for example, few drugs penetrate the blood-brain barrier.

DRUG SYNERGY

As in antibiotic therapy, the combination of two drugs may lead to synergy, where drugs are antagonistic to each other for various reasons.

PHARMACOLOGY OF CYTOTOXIC DRUGS

The five main classes of drugs will be discussed.

Alkylating Agents

By binding to guanine bases on separate strands of the DNA chain, alkylating agents form bridges between the strands and prevent them from separating at the time of DNA replication.

Common examples: Cyclophosphamide, Chlorambucil, Melphalan, Busulphan.

Anti-metabolites

These are compounds that are structurally similar (analogs) to the normal metabolites of the cell, which are required for cell function and replication. They are, however, functionally different, and if a high concentration is present in the cell, the drug will be taken up by the enzymes rather than the natural metabolite.

Common examples: Methotrexate, 6-Mercaptopurine, Thioguanine, 5-Fluorouracil, Cytosine Arabinoside, 5-Azacytidine.

Vinca Alkaloids

Vinca alkaloids are derived from the periwinkle plant, *Vinca major*. They are mitotic inhibitors, and are thought to interfere with nucleic acid synthesis at the metaphase stage.

Common examples: Vincristine, Vinblastine.

Antimitotic Antibiotics

These drugs inhibit tumour cell division in a way similar to the bactericidal action of antibiotics. They interfere with cellular metabolism in widely differing ways.

Common examples: Actinomycin D, Bleomycin, Adriamycin, Daunorubicin.

Miscellaneous Drugs (which do not fit into the above categories)

The nitrosoureas (BCNU, CCNU) and cis-platinum have some alkylating activity but have additional cytotoxic mechanisms. L-asparaginase depletes the body pool of asparagine, which is an essential amino acid. Normal cells can synthesise their own asparagine, whereas malignant cells cannot, and therefore die. Asparaginase is the only cytotoxic drug that preferentially kills tumour cells.

SIDE-EFFECTS OF DRUGS

Unfortunately, cytotoxic drugs are not selective, and, therefore, have a toxic effect on all rapidly dividing cells. It is for this reason that the hair follicles, the lining of the gastrointestinal tract and the bone marrow are the main focus for unpleasant side-effects.

Hair follicles

Hair loss (alopecia) is distressing for all members of the family, and it is little reassurance to tell them that the hair will eventually grow back (see Figure 5.3).

Gastrointestinal tract

Many cytotoxic drugs cause nausea and vomiting due to their effect on the central nervous system, whether it be a direct effect or anticipatory. The most useful anti-emetics are those with a sedative action, but on the whole are unsuccessful in completely alleviating it. Relaxation with visual imagery has been found to be helpful in the treatment of anticipatory vomiting (Morrow and Morrell, 1982). Nabilone (a synthetic form of cannabis) has recently been found to be a useful anti-emetic, but must be commenced before therapy (see Figure 5.3). Diarrhoea is common when drugs affect the large bowel. Septicaemia can occur when the integrity of the gut is compromised. Constipation is a common side-effect of the vinca alkaloids (see Figure 5.3). Stomatitis can be very debilitating for a child and should be avoided if at all possible (see Figure 5.3).

Generally, children receive good dental care and have healthy mouths so do not suffer severe problems. There are, however, some drugs which cause unavoidable toxicity to the oral mucosa.

Examples: High-dose Methotrexate, High-dose Melphalan.

Scrupulous mouth care will help to alleviate symptoms and Difflam has been found to relieve discomfort. A dry mouth is a

Figure 5.3 Care plan for a child receiving chemotherapy, using Henderson's model of nursing

NURSING CARE PLAN   CASE NO.   SHEET NO.

Patient's Name ....

Date	No.	Problem/Need	Goal	Action to be taken (Please sign each entry)	Review Date	Evaluation (Please date and sign each entry)

Core Care Plan for a Child Receiving Chemotherapy using Henderson's Model of Nursing

HNI = Henderson's Need Identified   PPA = Patient Problems Arising

1. Breathe. 2. Eat and drink. 3. Eliminate. 4. Move and maintain desirable posture. 5. Sleep and rest. 6. Select suitable clothing. 7. Maintain body temperature. 8. Keep body clean. 9. Avoid dangers in environment/avoid injuries. 10. Communicate. 11. Worship. 12. Work at something. 13. Play or participate in recreation. 14. Learn, discover or satisfy curiosity.

HNI (9)	PPA (1)	Potential infection May be neutropenic as a result of chemotherapy	Early detection of infection and prevention of cross infection	– 4-hourly observations of temperature, pulse and respirations – Report any changes to nurse in charge – Inspect skin for signs of infection twice daily (a) observe site of i.v. cannulae (b) inspect perianal area – Change giving sets daily – If child becomes neutropenic, nurse in protective isolation in cubicle – Change all linen and gowns daily – Damp dust cubicle daily		

Date	No.	Problem/Need	Goal	Action to be taken (Please sign each entry)	Review Date	Evaluation (Please date and sign each entry)
HNI (9)	PPA (2)	Potential bleeding Platelet count may be low as a result of chemotherapy	To detect bleeding	– 4-hourly observations of pulse and respirations – Report a rapid, thready pulse to nurse in charge – Test all urine, stools and vomit for blood – Observe for petechiae, bruises and frank bleeding – Take care with i.m. injections – Do not give Aspirin – Brush teeth with a small, soft brush, e.g. size 10		
HNI (9)	PPA (3)	Tiredness, lethargy, irritability, caused by low haemoglobin	To detect low haemoglobin	– Observe for pallor or lethargy – Observe for frank blood loss – Report a rapid, thready pulse to nurse in charge		
HNI (2)	PPA (4)	Potential sore mouth as a result of chemotherapy	To prevent infection and allow good diet and fluid intake	– Inspect mouth daily for signs of infection, ulcers and bleeding – Give extra fluids, or rinse mouth with water – Encourage tooth brushing with a good soft brush after meals and at bedtime. – Give well-diluted mouth washes if infection present – Apply Vaseline if lips are dry and cracked – Prophylactic Nystatin suspension to be prescribed if neutropenic and/or Candida present		

(Figure 5.3, continued)

Date	No.	Problem/Need	Goal	Action to be taken (Please sign each entry)	Review Date	Evaluation (Please date and sign each entry)
HNI (3)	PPA (5)	Potential bowel changes as a result of chemotherapy Diarrhoea and constipation	To monitor bowel actions and pre-empt complications	– Record all bowel actions on chart – Observe stool and test for blood – Report any diarrhoea or rectal bleeding to nurse in charge – If child is constipated give laxatives as prescribed to avoid complications and perianal fissures		
HNI (2)	PPA (6)	Potential anorexia as a result of chemotherapy	To monitor weight and pre-empt severe weight loss	– Weigh Monday, Wednesday and Friday – Encourage high-calorie nutritious diet – Encourage high-calorie nutritious drinks if child is unwilling to eat – Suggest parents provide food to child's liking – Enlist help of dietitian if necessary		
HNI (2)	PPA (7)	Potential nausea and vomiting as a result of chemotherapy	To relieve nausea and prevent vomiting To maintain adequate nutrition	– Give regular anti-emetics as prescribed – Warn child (as appropriate) and parents that anti-emetics may make them feel sleepy or 'high' – Reassure patient and parents. Aim to get them to relax as much as possible – Ensure clean vomit bowl and tissues are always available – Rinse mouth frequently to clear debris		

Date	No.	Problem/Need	Goal	Action to be taken (Please sign each entry)	Review Date	Evaluation (Please date and sign each entry)
HNI (10)	PPA (8)	Low morale as a result of anxiety, fear and isolation	To boost morale and relieve anxiety as much as possible	– Encourage parents to be resident and assist with the care of their child – Spend time with child and parents – allow them to talk and express their fears and anxieties – Ensure the child and parents are told of all treatment, tests and investigations – Explain plans to them as many times as necessary – Ensure that siblings are involved with the child		
HNI (13)	PPA (9)	Boredom due to isolation from home environment	To relieve boredom and provide suitable diversions	– Involve play therapist in therapeutic play programme – Provide diversions		
HNI (6)	PPA (10)	Alopecia and altered body image	To prepare child for potential hair loss and relieve anxiety as far as possible	– Explain to child and parents that hair will fall out – Arrange for child to have a wig if necessary or suggest that child wears knitted hats, scarves, baseball caps, etc. – Give reassurance that hair will grow back again		
HNI (11)	PPA (11)	Potential needle phobia due to repeated cannulation	To relieve distress	– Aim to take child's mind off procedure – Explain reason why it must be performed – Enlist help of psychologist to teach relaxation and meditation		

breeding ground for infection, and it should be rinsed with water as often as possible. Commercial mouth washes must be well diluted and used with caution, as they can be very drying to the oral mucosa. Glycerin and lemon, because of its hygroscopic action, can also be very drying and is not recommended. Sodium bicarbonate (a teaspoonful to 1 pint water) or normal saline (1 teaspoonful to 1 pint water) are used to clear debris from the mouth. Cotton buds or gauze wrapped around the finger are best suited for this purpose – forceps should never be used. Children very soon learn how to care for their own mouths and become very proficient.

Bone Marrow

The arrest of stem cell division in the bone marrow causes immunosuppression and neutropenia (granulocytes have a life-span of less than one week), and the child is therefore prone to infection (see Figure 5.3). Platelet counts may also fall rapidly, requiring replacement transfusions (see Figure 5.3).

Measles and chicken-pox pose a particular threat to immuno-suppressed children. It is therefore vital to give human immune globulin (HIG) and zoster immune globulin (ZIG) if the child has not had the disease and has been in direct contact with it. Since the introduction of acyclovir, an anti-viral agent, deaths due to disseminated chicken-pox have been almost eliminated. Measles, however, remains a fatal disease in some of these children.

Pneumocystis carinii and cytomegalovirus (CMV) can also be life-threatening. Prophylactic Septrin may be given to prevent pneumocystis pneumonia and high-dose Septrin would be given for an overt infection. CMV can be acquired naturally, like glandular fever, or can be transmitted by blood products from donors who have had the infection themselves. Screening of all blood products is undertaken to prevent CMV. This is not necessary if the child has already been exposed to the virus (CMV + ve). Children who are immunosuppressed should not receive any live virus immunisations during chemotherapy and for one year afterwards.

Needle phobia

Needle phobia can become a very real problem for a child receiving repeated venepunctures, and apart from the acute pain of such procedures seems to be associated with a fear of being attacked and having no control over it. Cytotoxic drugs produce unpleasant side-effects and it is therefore not surprising that some children are actually afraid that they are being given the drugs as some sort of punishment. Central venous lines are a major breakthrough for these children and in some cases it is feasible to keep them in situ for the total duration of treatment. Emla cream (lignocaine 25 mg and prilocaine 25 mg/g), a topical anaesthetic, sometimes helps by relieving pain, and relaxation with visual imagery has proved useful for adolescents (Hilgard and Le Baron, 1982).

Allowing a child to administer his own treatment may help to alleviate some of his fears, but must be strictly supervised.

Long-term Side-effects

Although the side-effects described above are common to most cytotoxic agents, many have their own toxic effects which should be mentioned. Bleomycin, for example, can cause irreversible lung fibrosis. Frequent administration of vinca alkaloids can cause peripheral neuropathy. The anthracyclines (Daunorubicin and Adriamycin) may cause cumulative cardiac damage (Praga et al, 1979); cis-platinum is oto- and nephrotoxic. High-dose cyclophosphamide can cause chemical cystitis. Most effects are related to the cumulative dose of the drug and careful screening before and during treatment allows modifications to be made, if necessary.

As patients survive longer, the late effects of chemotherapy are being revealed (Ferguson, 1981). Endocrine function and fertility may be reduced by certain forms of treatment and alkylating agents in particular can induce permanent sterility in males (Sherins et al, 1978). The alkylating agents, although useful, appear to be a contributory factor towards the development of second malignancies (Shalot et al, 1977).

NURSING CARE

It can be seen that the major side-effects of cytotoxic drugs present a unique challenge to nursing care. This is described in detail on Figure 5.3.

The predetermined sample care nursing plan (Glasper et al, 1987) is based on Virginia Henderson's conceptual framework. All the care problems are referenced to Henderson's fourteen activities of daily living (HNI). Henderson's framework has been chosen because many nurses feel comfortable with it. It is, however, the responsibility of the primary nurse to decide which model is most appropriate for her use. The Core Care Plan has identified key problems shared by all children receiving chemotherapy. Clearly, a full assessment must be made and individual problems added to complete the care plan.

CLINICAL TRIALS

The dramatic improvement in treatment for children with cancer has been largely due to cooperative studies by the United Kingdom Children's Cancer Study Group (UKCCSG) or controlled clinical trials run in this country by the Medical Research Council.

Permission to enter patients into these trials is sought from the local Ethical Committee and informed consent obtained from parents. It is often difficult to explain to parents the efficacy of clinical trials if randomisation is used. It is, however, important to explain carefully the rationale behind such trials and the subsequent success, as a result of their use.

ROUTES OF ADMINISTRATION

Intravenous Route

Many cytotoxic drugs are given by the intravenous route to maximise their therapeutic effect. Most of these agents are potentially sclerosing, and safe administration to children who cannot appreciate the importance of keeping limbs still and who are poorly supplied with peripheral veins, can pose great practical difficulties.

The use of central venous lines has revolutionised intravenous therapy, especially when children are to receive many courses of treatment (Figure 5.4). The catheter is usually inserted into the subclavian vein, under general anaesthetic. It is tunnelled under the skin of the chest and brought to the surface some distance from the vein. Awareness of the potential risk of infection or air embolism should be an overriding factor in deciding local policy for care of these lines.

More recently, totally implantable devices with self-sealing diaphragms have been used in some centres. They are cosmetically more pleasing and allow greater mobility, but these advantages may be outweighed by their expense and the discomfort of multiple-needle punctures to obtain access to the reservoir. Emla cream has been found to be effective for children receiving venepunctures and may be effective in this case also.

Venepunctures should be performed using a strict aseptic technique. The site should be carefully chosen and the cannula taped securely without covering the puncture site.

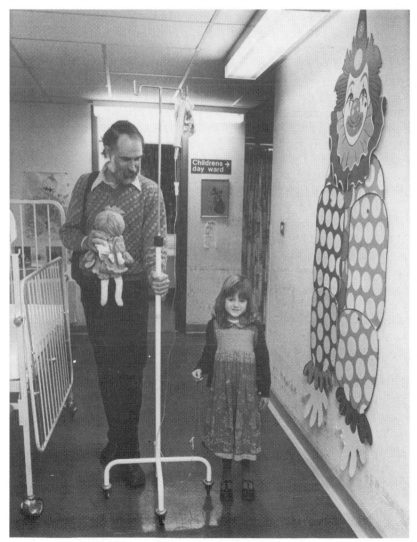

Figure 5.4   With a central venous catheter in situ,
the child has greater freedom

Intrathecal Route

This route is used to treat or prevent central nervous system disease in leukaemia or lymphoma. Methotrexate is most commonly used, but the dose is limited, due to the risk of neurological and systemic toxicity.

Intramuscular Route

Cytosine arabinoside is sometimes given by the intramuscular route; this does not appear to pose a problem.

Asparaginase is used to treat acute lymphatic leukaemia. This drug can cause an acute anaphylactic reaction. It is therefore essential that hydrocortisone, chlorpheniramine and adrenaline are to hand and medical assistance is readily available. The child is quite likely to have a low platelet count at the time of administration, and it is important to minimise trauma to the tissues as far as is possible.

Oral Route

Drugs administered by the oral route usually cause fewer immediate side-effects. Tablets may be crushed or capsules may need to be broken open for younger children. It is best to avoid the latter if possible because the contents of capsules can be very irritant to the mouth and may cause ulceration. The hands should be protected and a mask worn if capsules are opened as it is easy to inhale the powder. Some drugs should be taken on an empty stomach for maximum absorption. Parents may need to be reminded of this.

Hazards

The potential hazards associated with the administration of cytotoxic drugs should be taken seriously by all concerned with their use. They can be mutagenic, carcinogenic and probably teratogenic (Williams, 1985; Sherry et al, 1985). They can be absorbed through the skin and mucous membranes, which in itself can cause irritation; and leakage of a drug into the tissues can cause severe necrosis (Smith, 1985). The administration of cytotoxic agents, therefore, should be undertaken by a specialist nurse who has received appropriate instruction (Marks, 1981).

The three guiding principles behind cytotoxic drug preparation and administration are to protect the handler, the environment and the patient.

Protection of the Handler

Protective clothing, PVC (Trifix) gloves and goggles should be worn. If a drug accidentally comes in contact with the skin or eyes it should be washed off with cold running water and reported immediately. To avoid needle stick injuries, needles should not be replaced in plastic sheaths after use but should be disposed of in a 'sharps' container. Masks need only be worn if loose powder is being reconstituted.

Protection of the Environment

Ideally, cytotoxic drugs should be prepared in a laminar flow cabinet. If this is impossible, a well-ventilated room, removed from the mainstream of staff and patients, should be used. Spillage should be wiped up immediately; working over a tray helps to contain this. The use of filters avoids aerosol sprays. Protective sheaths should be left on needles when expelling air.

Glass ampoules should be broken, using a swab to avoid cuts and spillage.

All materials used should be disposed of, taking great care to avoid contamination.

Protection of the Patient

It is frightening for a child and indeed many adults to be approached by a nurse wearing full protective clothing. It is therefore advisable to wear PVC gloves only. Drugs should be given slowly into a fast-flowing drip. If a peripheral vein is used, great care should be taken to ensure that the cannula is in the vein, and that no extravasation is occurring. The line should be well flushed after use. Medical advice should be sought if extravasation is suspected.

The skin should be protected at the site of administration, and the point of access should be as far away from the patient as possible.

The above are only guidelines, and it is up to each unit to provide a local policy.

COPING WITH CHEMOTHERAPY

The Child

The cure rate for childhood cancer has increased dramatically, but a price has to be paid in terms of concomitant toxicity.

The debilitating side-effects of chemotherapy pose an enormous threat to the body image and self-control of a child, especially if he is an adolescent.

Despite efforts to promote adequate nutrition, nausea, vomiting, anorexia, diarrhoea and stomatitis are likely to cause cachexia and weight loss.

Hair loss, in addition to being traumatic for the child, undoubtedly changes his appearance.

It is therefore little wonder that it is so difficult for the older child to return to school, especially when he is also probably feeling tired and perhaps a little unwell. However, despite these limitations, it is undoubtedly beneficial for the child to return to school, because it is his link with normality. His uncertainty will be allayed if the school personnel understand what is expected of them (Ackerman et al, 1986) and his peers appreciate the importance of their support. Most children on chemotherapy are able to join in games and take part in all school activities; and it is important to ensure that we bend the rules governing treatment plans to allow them to do this. With this in mind, day care for children receiving chemotherapy should be encouraged. It allows a more flexible approach and the child does not suffer the inevitable trauma of feeling 'hospitalised'.

Understanding children's views of treatment is an important part of delivering effective care. For younger children, the threat and pain of intrusive procedures are feared more than the disease itself. Honest and appropriate information and preparation should be provided, according to the age and maturity of the child. Play therapy is an invaluable tool to instruct the younger child.

Siblings

Sibling too must cope with childhood cancer and all that is associated with it. No matter how careful parents are, siblings usually feel left out and may suffer in later years as a result (Doyle, 1987).

Parents

Coping with childhood cancer is not easy for any member of the family. How, then, can we as nurses help parents gain the strength to cope? For cope they must if the child is to undergo treatment in order to effect a cure (Evans, 1987).

There are three key ingredients to assist parents to regain control so that they are better able to cope.

Information

Parents and, indeed, children require knowledge; this must be tailored to individual needs. They need to know how chemotherapy works, what side-effects to expect and what the protocol entails. Written information helps to reinforce verbal information, and gives families time to digest it. Fear of the unknown and a vivid imagination can cause untold damage.

Support

The conflict between exposing your child to toxic chemotherapy or allowing him to die seems easy to resolve. When faced with this conflict, however, parents suffer enormous stress and each new 'assault' on their child seems to threaten their stability. Hair loss is one example of this, and the parents usually suffer much more than the child. Parents, then, need to know that staff are available, that they are prepared to listen in an effort to be sensitive to how they are feeling. To achieve this effectively, staff too need support, otherwise they are ineffective and become 'burnt-out'.

Meticulous Nursing Care

Attention to detail and anticipation of potential problems are the essence of the nursing care of patients receiving chemotherapy. To involve parents in the care of their children may be the only way to achieve this, but as long as they are well supervised, it must surely be to everyone's advantage.

CONCLUSION

Our aim is to cure childhood cancer; chemotherapy is our most effective weapon at present. And, if in the end a child must die, at least we can prolong his survival and offer him a reasonable quality of life.

References

Ackerman J, Dutton S, Evans M and Johnson C (1986) *The Child with Cancer in School*. Wessex: Wessex Cancer Trust.

Doyle B (1987) I wish you were dead. *Nursing Times*, **83**(45): 44–46.

Evans M (1987) Learning to lose fear. *Nursing Times*, **83**(17): 55–56.

Ferguson J H (1981) Cognitive late effects of treatment for acute lymphocytic leukaemia in childhood. *Topics in Clinical Nursing*, **2**: 21–29.

Glasper A, Stonehouse J and Martin L (1987) Core care plans. *Nursing Times*, **83**(10): 55–57.

Hilgard J and Le Baron S (1982) Relief of anxiety and pain in children and adolescents with cancer: quantitive measure and clinical observations. *Journal of Clinical and Experimental Hypnosis*, **XXX:** 417–442.

Marks M (1981) Intravenous therapy: the extended role of the nurse. *Nursing Focus*, **8**(11): 377–381.

Morrow G R and Morrell C (1982) Behavioural treatment for anticipatory nausea and vomiting induced by cancer chemotherapy. *New England Journal of Medicine*, **307**: 1476–1480.

Praga C, Beretta G, Vigo P L et al (1979) Adriamycin cardiotoxicity: a survey of 1273 patients. *Cancer Treatment Reports*, **63**(5): 827–834.

Shalot S M, Beardwell C G, Twomay J A, Morris Jones P H and Pearson D (1977) Endocrine function following the treatment of A.L.L. in childhood. *Journal of Paediatrics*, **90**: 920–923.

Sherins R J, Olwery C L M and Ziegler J L (1978) Gynecomastia and gonadal dysfunction in adolescent boys treated with combination chemotherapy for Hodgkin's disease. *New England Journal of Medicine*, **299**: 12–16.

Sherry G et al (1985) A study of occupational exposure to antineoplastic drugs and foetal loss in nurses. *New England Journal of Medicine*, **313**(19): 1173–1177.

Smith R (1985) Prevention and treatment of extravasation. *British Journal of Parenteral Therapy*, **6**(5): 114–118.

Williams C J (1985) Handling cytotoxics. *British Medical Journal*, **291**: 1299–1300.

Further Reading

Cancer Chemotherapy, Eli Lilly Oncology Service.

Carter S K, Bahowski M T and Hellmann K (1981) *Chemotherapy of Cancer*. New York: John Wiley and Sons.

Green J A, Macbeth F R and Williams C J (1983) *Medical Oncology*. Oxford: Blackwell Scientific Publications.

Priestman T J (1977) *Cancer Chemotherapy: an Introduction.* Herts: Montedison Pharmaceuticals.

Skeel R T (ed.) (1982) *Manual of Cancer Chemotherapy.* Boston: Little, Brown.

APPENDIX
NEW APPROACHES TO THERAPY

Many tumours show a dose-response relation to cytotoxic drugs, but the amount of drug that can be given is limited mainly by the toxic effect on the bone marrow. If this can be circumvented by the replacement of haemopoietic stem cells following ablative therapy, the dosage of drugs can be raised by a factor of 3.

If a small percentage of the patient's own bone marrow is removed prior to high-dose therapy and subsequently reinfused, the term autologous bone marrow transplant or autograft is used. In an allogeneic transplant, or allograft, marrow is donated from a histocompatible sibling. In both cases, marrow is harvested by multiple aspirations from the iliac bones, but can be reinfused intravenously and will return to the marrow.

In paediatric practice, allogeneic transplants are now recommended for children with acute myeloid leukaemia, and in some cases of 'high-risk' or relapsed lymphoblastic leukaemia. Autografts have mainly been used for poor prognosis tumours such as neuroblastoma, or for children with leukaemia who have no histocompatible sibling.

The most exciting recent development in cancer therapy has been the introduction of techniques for targeting drugs or radiotherapy on a tumour. Monoclonal antibodies have been raised to a variety of tumours and can be chemically coupled to toxins or cytotoxic drugs. When injected into the patient, high doses of antibody-bound drug can be given since it targets on the tumour cells with sparing of normal tissues. Initial results are encouraging. Monoclonal antibodies can also be linked to radioactive compounds, such as iodine 131 and used to stage and sometimes treat certain tumours. As more specific antibodies become available, targeting techniques should advance so that drugs can be used to maximum effect with minimum side-effects.

Acknowledgements

My grateful thanks to Dr Jan Kohler for her valuable advice and for so willingly writing the Appendix on 'New Approaches to Therapy' and to Alan Glasper, Lecturer in Paediatric Nursing Studies, and Staff Nurse Susan Moore for their help in the care plan.

Many thanks also to the Wessex Cancer Trust for their support.

6
The Child Receiving Radiotherapy

INTRODUCTION

Radiotherapy is an important component of treatment for children with cancer. The practicalities of treatment have changed little over the past twenty years, although the machines have become more powerful (James, 1985). People may have unfounded ideas about radiotherapy: Eardley (1986) states that 43 per cent of patients in the adult institution expected the treatment to be painful. It is important that parents and children do not have such misapprehensions and that they understand what to expect before treatment begins.

WHAT IS RADIOTHERAPY?

There are two types of ionising radiation used for treatment:

- Electromagnetic (X-rays and gamma rays)
- Particulate (neutrons, alpha and beta particles).

X-rays are by definition manmade. Gamma rays are similar but are produced by the breakdown of radioactive isotopes such as cobalt or radium. X-rays are produced by the acceleration of electrons onto a target, usually tungsten, which absorbs the energy, producing heat and electromagnetic radiation. Low-energy X-rays are used for conventional diagnostic purposes. High-energy X-rays, produced by linear accelerators, are used for treatment. The amount of radiation energy absorbed by body tissues is measured in *grays*.

A beam of X-rays ionises whatever lies in its path in a random manner. Damage to ribonucleic acid (RNA) and deoxyribonucleic acid (DNA) is the most significant consequence of radiotherapy and occurs in different ways: firstly, by damage to purine and especially pyrimidine bases (cytosine, thymine, and uracil); secondly, by single and double helix strand breaks. Such damage will not usually immediately kill a cell. Only when the time comes for cell division will the damage be revealed; mitosis will fail and the cell then dies. Proliferating normal cells such as bone marrow or gut epithelium show the effects of radiation rapidly and are said to be 'radiosensitive'. The more rapid the turnover, the more sensitive the tissue. Non-proliferating tissues, on the other hand, such as neurones, are relatively radioresistant. Small blood vessels have intermediate sensitivity but damage to them may lead to the anoxic death of some dependent radioresistant cells.

X-rays produce lethal and sub-lethal damage in both tumours and normal tissues. The sub-lethal damage is repaired within a few hours. Lethal damage cannot be repaired although repopulation may occur from surrounding undamaged cells. Tumour cells are usually less efficient than normal tissues both in repairing sub-lethal damage and in repopulation.

Any tumour can theoretically be eradicated by radiation, but the dose required may cause unacceptable damage to normal tissue. In practice radiocurability therefore depends on the tolerance of normal tissue within the irradiated area. If a tumour is in a highly radiosensitive tissue, such as liver, this limits the amount of radiation that can safely be delivered. Thus radiation may not be an appropriate modality in this situation, i.e. the tumour may be radiosensitive but not radiocurable.

As a general rule the larger the neoplasm, the larger the dose required to control it. Larger tumours generally have a poor blood supply and their lack of oxygen makes them less sensitive to radiotherapy. In addition, the proportion of cells that are actually dividing is smaller.

Fractionation refers to the division of a total dose of radiotherapy into several treatments. Tumour cells repair sub-lethal damage between fractions but do this less efficiently than normal cells leading to an enhanced therapeutic ratio.

TREATMENT GROUPS

Radiotherapy is used to treat children for a variety of diseases and for different diagnoses within these diseases.

1. It forms part of the *primary treatment* of children with the following tumours:

   • Brain tumours
   • Rhabdomyosarcoma
   • Ewing's sarcoma

- Retinoblastoma
- Advanced stage Wilms' tumour
- Localised Hodgkin's disease

2. *Prophylaxis.* The central nervous system may act as a sanctuary site for leukaemia cells. Prevention of central nervous system relapse in treatment of acute lymphoblastic leukaemia in Great Britain is achieved with cranial irradiation, plus intrathecal methotrexate. This may present difficulties if a child has a later central nervous system relapse because of the damage which may be caused by irradiating the brain twice.

3. Children are *prepared* for allogenic bone marrow transplantation with total body irradiation, which has the dual purpose of killing residual malignant cells and normal marrow.

4. It has a *palliative* role especially in controlling pain in children for whom treatment has failed. The metastatic area can be irradiated, or, if metastases are extensive, hemi-body irradiation may be used. Good pain relief is obtained in most children, contributing to an improved quality of life.

SIDE-EFFECTS OF RADIOTHERAPY

Reactions to radiotherapy can be divided into three categories: acute, early delayed and the long-term.

Acute Reactions

Acute reactions may occur during the course of radiotherapy. Problems include vomiting, tiredness, and skin reaction around the site (Thomson, 1980; Holmes, 1986a). Vomiting, which has been dealt with elsewhere in this book, may be protracted for some children. The use of rectal phenothiazines may be appropriate. Children receiving treatment for brain tumours may suffer a transient increase in intracranial pressure, probably due to oedema. Steroids are frequently given to lessen this. Inflamed skin should, if possible, not be included in the radiation field because the situation may be exacerbated. However, topical steroids may be considered if the inflammation becomes severe and threatens the completion of radiotherapy.

Treated skin is also very sensitive to direct sunlight and should therefore be protected.

Early Delayed Reactions

Early delayed reactions occur soon after the treatment. Bone marrow depression may occur when the spine is treated. Hair loss will only occur when the head is included in the field. If the abdomen is included then nausea, vomiting and diarrhoea may occur. If large volumes of lung are treated, radiation pneumonitis may occur. When the salivary glands are included then parotitis is not uncommon with accompanying swelling and later xerostomia may occur. The advent of convenient artificial saliva sprays, especially those containing mucin, have helped to alleviate these problems, which include dry mouth causing difficulties with speech. The additions of liquids, e.g. gravy, cream or custard, may help the mouth during meals. It seems that it is the older child who suffers most, although this may only be because the problem can be articulated. Loss of taste may also occur. It is then even more difficult to persuade the child to eat. Problems with the mouth may lead to an unwillingness or inability to eat with consequent malnutrition. This needs to be anticipated and preventative measures taken, e.g. enteral feeding using long indwelling nasogastric tubes (Holmes, 1986b). If the lower gastrointestinal tract has been treated then there may occasionally be problems with mal-absorption. In some instances, such as the child with a rhabdomyosarcoma of the middle ear, when prolonged radio-therapy and chemotherapy will be required, a gastrostomy may be appropriate prior to radiation. It is likely that the more well nourished the child with cancer, the greater are the chances of becoming a long-term survivor.

Forward planning is also necessary with the dentition when the head is to be irradiated. Irradiated bone has a limited ability to repair itself or grow. Some authorities believe that potentially problematic teeth, such as wisdom teeth, should be removed before irradiation, especially as radiation necrosis is difficult to treat. Radiation-induced caries can be prevented by the education of parents and children. Frequent teeth cleaning and general oral hygiene, as well as dental checks, should be stressed. There is also a place for the use of stannous fluoride gel either alone or in trays (like a rugby player's gum shield).

Other problems include sleepiness, and lethargy in children receiving treatment to the brain, due to the temporary disruption of myelin formation. The symptoms usually last about two to three weeks and occur six to ten weeks after completion of treatment, corresponding to the length of time it takes for myelin repair. This is called the 'somnolence syndrome' and is a period which can be very worrying for parents if they are not forewarned. They should be told that the child may appear to 'hibernate' for two to three weeks. He may also feel very depressed during this period. Attempts have been made to alleviate these symptoms with prophylactic antidepressants in adults but are not of proven value and are little used in children.

Long-term Consequences

The long-term consequences centre on effects in the growth of bone and soft tissues and on endocrine glands, such as the pituitary, thyroid glands, the testes and ovaries (Brockbank and Hodgkinson, 1981).

Bone Growth

Bone which has been irradiated is unlikely to continue to grow. This causes an overall reduction in affected bone length. Growth in length of bone occurs at the epiphysis. The major contribution to a child's ultimate height comes from growth around the knee, i.e. at the distal end of the femur and the proximal end of the tibia. The other major growth area is the vertebral column. Any irradiation to these sites may result in diminished growth. Any asymmetric radiotherapy can also cause problems. If half the spine is irradiated, this can lead to a scoliosis (Mayfield, 1979). This occasionally occurred in the past during treatment for Wilms' tumour or neuroblastoma. Now it is standard practice for the whole width of the spine to be irradiated. Children who receive treatment to the head of femur were prone to develop slipped epiphysis, but it is now shielded where possible. The child's growth should be monitored carefully, keeping an accurate record of weight, standing and sitting height. Growth will be slowed down during treatment, whether by drugs or radiation, and children, especially the younger ones, are unlikely to regain their former positions on the centile chart. Their growth may be affected by their general condition, including their emotional and nutritional state.

Endocrine

Cranial irradiation, e.g. for brain tumours, can affect the pituitary gland. The production of growth hormone appears to be the most sensitive, but other pituitary hormones that may be affected are the gonadotrophins, adrenocortico-tropic hormone and thyroid stimulating hormone. Any irradiation to either the thyroid gland or gonads may also seriously affect these organs; the endocrinologist is therefore a valuable team member.

Continuous monitoring of growth with appropriate tests of pituitary function should identify those children who would benefit from replacement growth hormone at a stage early enough to allow them to obtain maximum benefit from it.

Children who receive radiotherapy to the neck are liable to thyroid dysfunction (Guimond, 1979). Some may require replacement thyroxine and their thyroid status needs to be monitored at regular intervals.

There is a large group of children who receive cranial irradiation for central nervous system prophylaxis during the treatment of acute lymphoblastic leukaemia. It is suggested that this may lead to an overall reduction in intelligence quotient (IQ) of ten points (Eiser and Lansdown, 1977; Moss et al, 1981; Twaddle et al, 1983). It may not be noticeable to the family, especially as the children are mostly under seven years of age during treatment, although it may become more obvious with time as the child's achievements are compared with his siblings and peers.

Radiotherapy to the whole abdomen or pelvis in females will have a detrimental effect upon the ovaries. There will be a reduction in secondary sexual characteristics, amenorrhoea and infertility. Oral oestrogen and progesterone replacement will help development of the secondary sexual characteristics and monthly cyclical use will induce menstrual bleeding. Oestrogen in particular aids vaginal lubrication and may well help to prevent long-term osteoporosis.

Testicular irradiation is now not commonly given; there was a phase in the development of treatment for acute lymphoblastic leukaemia when attempts were made to improve the poor prognosis for boys by giving a relatively low dose of prophy-lactic testicular irradiation. There are now many long-term survivors who although they have normal hormonal function of the testes are infertile. Higher doses of radiotherapy are given where there is definitive testicular disease and these boys may also have problems with testosterone production and require replacement therapy. However, it is important to ensure that the parents understand that although their son may be infertile, he should not be impotent. Adolescent boys presenting for the first time with cancer may be offered the opportunity to store semen in a sperm bank for use later in life after successful treatment of the cancer.

RADIOTHERAPY AND CHEMOTHERAPY

Before the advent of chemotherapy, radiation was often given as the only modality of treatment following surgery. However, there are very few instances now where radiotherapy is given without chemotherapy. Some drugs do interact and potentiate the effects of radiotherapy and careful thought needs to be given to these during the planning of protocols and their subsequent execution.

Certain drugs present specific difficulties. Actinomycin D, Adriamycin and bleomycin appear to be broad-spectrum augmentors of radiation effect (except to the brain and the eye). Together these treatments are more effective at killing cells than their theoretically combined effect. When these drugs are used after radiation is completed the radiation reaction can reappear and necrosis can occur. This is known as the 'recall' phenomenon. It is most noticeable when the skin becomes erythematous and desquamates within the former radiation field. Other difficulties relate to giving drugs with specific side-effects, e.g. Adriamycin and the heart. (When radiation is required to the heart, tolerance to Adriamycin is reduced.)

Hypoxic Cell Radiosensitisers

The core of a brain tumour, about 20 per cent of the cells, is hypoxic, and is not actively dividing or growing. These hypoxic cells are not effectively killed by irradiation. When radiation therapy is completed and the oxygenated cells are killed or fatally damaged, the hypoxic cells may then receive oxygen and divide. About three times the dose of radiation is required to kill hypoxic cells as opposed to oxygenated cells, but in some circumstances this dose might be lethal. To overcome the resistance of hypoxic cells, a class of drugs known as the nitroimidazoles is being tested, amongst these are metronidazole and misonidazole.

PREPARATION OF THE CHILD FOR TREATMENT

Radiotherapy is a frightening concept for most parents, whose only knowledge of it, if any, may be as a last chance treatment for an elderly relative. It cannot be seen and yet has profound effects. Treatment centres tend to be in large adult hospitals, where the majority of the treatment population is elderly. Despite the disproportionate efforts that radiotherapy staff make for the children, these institutions usually do not have a child-centred atmosphere.

Some families may have been referred to a number of different hospitals before they arrive at the regional children's cancer unit. Even though the diagnosis of cancer has been made, many express relief that they have discovered their child's problem. It is important that the radiotherapy institution be regarded as part of the organisation of the unit, rather than yet another place to be sent. Children receiving radiotherapy for central nervous system prophylaxis probably get the best service; they are approximately the same age, they receive the same treatment and they are numerous. This promotes good communication between parents, who help each other by telling them what to expect; they are in a unique position to do this. The remaining groups of children requiring radiotherapy tend to vary more by age and area to be irradiated (although brain tumours form a substantial treatment group). Professionals tend to be less familiar and, more obviously, parents are less likely to be supported by others in a similar position.

Various strategies have been adopted to solve these problems. Pamphlets have been produced to summarise treatment; these seem to be best when tailored to each institution. A pre-eminent example is the booklet produced by the University of Indiana (Dudjak, 1987). This gives clear explanations about treatment and side-effects, and allows parents to ask about side-effects that their child might suffer. Adding actual photographs of the treatment rooms, waiting rooms and the hospital will help both the parent and child to have a better understanding of where they are going. Photographs of the actual personnel involved may be even better. Nottingham have taken a different step and have produced a video about radiotherapy aimed at children, showing the treatment area. Nothing can substitute for a visit to the radiotherapy unit prior to the commencement of treatment and it would be good to see an increase in the number of children visiting before their trip for treatment planning. The goal of this visit would be to familiarise the child and family with the treatment room, the equipment, personnel and the procedure.

HANDLING THE CHILD THROUGH TREATMENT

Before Treatment

The treatment has initially to be 'planned' to ensure that the required volume is accurately treated and all surrounding structures are spared as much as possible. Children are given a test dose before the treatment starts. Recordings are taken of the ouput and the settings altered accordingly. The child may find that he is being surrounded by gel bags or similar. These are tissue-equivalent and allow the radiotherapist to change the effective shape of the child so that it is near to an easily calculable form, such as a rectangle. Sensitive structures such as the eye or lungs may be shielded and special lead blocks may be made for this purpose. These are attached to the machine, so that the metal creates a 'shadow' where no radiation will enter.

The child may need to be marked with dye so that the treatment can be lined up consistently. Part of the reason for not washing the irradiated area is to preserve these marks so that the treatment is accurate. It is often said that children must not wash during treatment; the reasons given are that the water will predispose to a skin reaction or the indelible marks identifying the treatment area may be washed off. It is impractical for a child not to wash during the period of radiotherapy. The important point is to inform the child and his family that no perfumed soaps, powders or ointments containing zinc or lead base should be used as these increase the sensitivity to irradiation. Water can be used and the area treated dabbed dry with a soft towel. Some baby powders and soaps can be used but should be checked before use.

The child with a brain tumour may require a fitted helmet to be made, usually of perspex. Unfortunately, the child has to have a plaster of Paris cast made first and the head may need to be greased beforehand. The technicians who do this are highly skilled and spend a great deal of time with the children to obtain a good fit. They have to come back to see that the helmet fits properly and more importantly, that they can cope with wearing it. These helmets then allow for accurate alignment of treatment and may also carry 'shields'. There is a trend to allow the children to keep them after treatment and some get worn as space helmets.

During Treatment

Unlike almost every other procedure that the child with cancer will face, radiation is the one that they have to face alone and in addition stay perfectly still. It would be dangerous for the parent to be with the child; this is dealt with in a variety of ways. Treatment times are usually only a few minutes. Some centres have mirrors or thickened lead glass, so that the children can see out and the parents can see in. Most have some form of intercom and some even have television cameras, to which some children respond well.

Despite these devices and the best efforts of all involved, it is sometimes necessary for the younger child to be anaesthetised for the procedure (Figure 6.1). This provides practical difficulties for the anaesthetist, because he is physically separated from the child. Leads are usually attached to the child and his respiration, heart rate and occasionally blood oxygen levels are monitored outside the treatment room. Speed reduces the obvious risk as does having an experienced paedriatric anaesthetist. (Ketamine is the anaesthetic agent frequently used because of its short duration of action.) It is common practice to use this anaesthetic to give intrathecal methotrexate during the

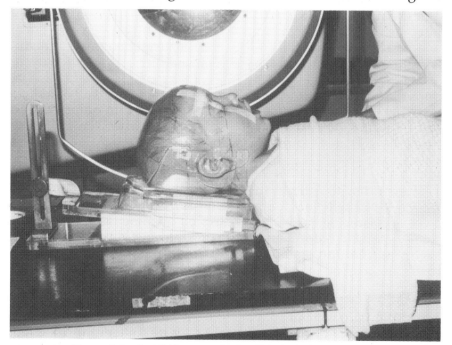

Figure 6.1   A child is anaesthetised for cranial radiotherapy

central nervous system prophylaxis phase of treatment of acute lymphoblastic leukaemia.

Family Involvement

Some radiotherapy treatments can last for several weeks. If the child is an in-patient with family far away, this can be a great strain. As the treatment lasts for only a few minutes each day some parents will prefer to travel daily, even considerable distances, so that they can be at home most of the time. This daily travelling can be a great strain on families both physically, emotionally and financially. As with all hospitalisation of children, siblings are likely to imagine terrible things happening to their brother or sister, or be jealous because they think that the other parent and child have gone on holiday. Letting the siblings visit the hospital to see the child and the treatment area will help to deal with this. If the child is coping well with radiotherapy, then weekend leave may be appropriate. If the child cannot be discharged home at all, then it may be possible to accommodate the whole family over weekends. However, these parents also need time for each other, so encouragement to grandparents, other relatives or a well-loved friend of the family to stay with the child may help the parents to cope.

NEW AND FUTURE TREATMENTS

Various new treatments are under study (Association for Brain Tumour Research, 1985) and could find their way to British paediatric oncology treatment protocols in the future.

Fast Neutron Radiation

Fast neutron radiation is less dependent on cells being well oxygenated. Because fast neutrons are also more damaging to normal tissues as well as tumour cells, it has been difficult to determine dosages. These tests are underway in Cyclotron facilities in the United States and Europe.

Hyperthermia

Hyperthermia has long been known to kill both normal and malignant cells. Because it would be lethal to heat up the entire body to the required temperatures, a new technique is being tested that will heat the tumour alone. For brain tumours a small hole is made in the skull and a rod or seed is implanted into the tumour. Using microwaves, ultrasound or radio waves, heat is generated by vibration. Because the centre of the tumour has no blood flow, the tumour cannot be cooled effectively, and the heat can therefore kill the malignant cells.

Interstitial Radiation

Interstitial radiation (brachytherapy) involves the placing of a source of radiation directly into the tumour rather than aiming waves of energy at it from ouside the body. The effect on normal tissue can be reduced while delivering a larger dose to the tumour itself. For this type of treatment to be effective, the tumour must be quite small (less than 5 cm in diameter). By emitting a continuous low dose of radiation to a tumour, oxygenation can continue, thus making the cells radiosensitive. Depending on the isotope, or seed implanted, treatment usually lasts from a few to several days. Steroids are commonly used with this therapy to reduce oedema. Unlike external radiation the patient is radioactive until the seed or implant is removed, and precautions are taken to protect those around him or her.

Targeted Radiotherapy

It has long been the dream of doctors treating cancer to have a 'magic bullet' which would treat cancer cells only and leave normal cells unaffected. For many years this approach has been used to treat thyroid cancer in adults and occasionally in children where a radioisotope, e.g. iodine 101, is given which is taken up specifically by the thyroid gland and releases its radiation within cells thus destroying them. However, this approach also kills normal thyroid cells. More recently attempts have been made to find substances which will be specifically taken up only by tumour cells. Again, a radioisotope, usually iodine 101, is attached to the substance and is released within or around the tumour cell. Antibodies specific to cancer cells are being developed. MIBG, a substance which is specifically taken up by tumours of the adrenal glands, e.g. neuroblastoma, is currently under investigation and good responses to treatment have been seen.

Radiotherapy is playing a decreasing role in the management of children with cancer. The recognition of the late effects of radiotherapy and the development of more effective chemotherapy regimes have resulted in this decline. However, it does still have an important and curative role for some malignancies and the radiotherapy team, both radiotherapists and radiographers, are important members of the paediatric oncology team. It is important to remember that the radiographers often get very emotionally attached to children whom they are treating and follow-up information should be relayed to them. An invitation should be extended to radiographers to attend long-term follow-up clinics to see the children who are well and leading normal lives many years after successful treatment.

References

Association for Brain Tumour Research (1985) *Treatment of Brain Tumours.* Chicago: A F B T R.

Brockbank P A and Hodgkinson S (1981) Long-term side-effects of radiotherapy in children. *Nursing Times*, **77**(50): 2152-2156.

Dudjak L A (1987) Radiation therapy: teaching the paediatric patient and the family. *Journal of the Association of Paediatric Oncology Nurses*, 4(1&2): 45-47.

Eardley A (1986) What do patients need to know? *Nursing Times*, **82**(17): 24-26.

Eiser C and Lansdown R (1977) Retrospective study of intellectual development in children treated for Acute Lymphoblastic Leukaemia. *Archives of Disease in Childhood*, **52**(7): 525-529.

Guimond J H (1979) Post-irradiation thyroid disorders. *American Journal of Nursing*, **79**(7): 1256-1258.

Holmes S (1986a) Radiotherapy, minimising the side effects. *Senior Nurse*, **1**(10): 263-265.

Holmes S (1986b) Planning nutritional support. *Nursing Times*, **82**(17): 26-29.

James R D (1985) Modern radiotherapy. *Update*, **31**(4): 829-844.

Mayfield J K (1979) Post radiational spine deformity. *Orthopaedic Clinics of North America*, **10**(4): 829-844.

Moss M H, Nannis E D and Poplack D G (1981) The effects of the prophylactic treatment of the central nervous system on the intellectual functioning of children with acute lymphocytic leukaemia. *American Journal of Medicine*, **71**(7): 47-52.

Thomson L (1980) Side effects of radiotherapy. *Nursing Times*, **76**(20): 877-881.

Twaddle V, Britton P G, Craft A C, Noble T C and Kernahan J (1983) Intellectual function after treatment for leukaemia or solid tumours. *Archives of Disease in Childhood*, **58**(12): 949-952.

7

The Child and Surgery

THE PLACE OF SURGERY IN PAEDIATRIC ONCOLOGY

Before 1950 radical surgery was the only treatment available for cancer. It was very rare for a child with cancer to be cured. With the introduction of chemotherapy and radiotherapy cure rates have improved and treatment by surgery alone has become less common. Ironically, it is the success of these other forms of treatment, as well as improvements in surgical techniques, which have led to the greater use of surgery in the management of paediatric malignancy.

The child with a malignant tumour that would previously have been described as 'inoperable' may now have a future if he receives appropriate combinations of therapy. It must be remembered that surgery and radiotherapy excluding total body irradiation are local treatments, whereas chemotherapy is systemic. So the importance of a multidisciplinary approach cannot be overstated. In some cases the surgeon will be involved at diagnosis and should not attempt biopsy or the removal of a suspected tumour without consulting other members of the oncology team.

Indications for Surgery

The place of surgery will differ in the management of each child, as well as in each type of malignancy. Figure 7.1 gives a

- Diagnosis and staging
- Treatment: emergency
                1 excision   – complete
                                      – partial
                delayed   – 1 excision
                                      – 2nd look
                excision of metastases
- Complication relief
- Symptom relief
- Vascular and intrathecal access

Figure 7.1   The place of surgery in paediatric oncology

guide to the situations where surgery may be considered as part of the overall treatment plan.

Diagnosis and Staging

With modern X-ray imaging and other tests, some childhood cancers can be diagnosed without histological examination of affected tissue. But using a surgical biopsy to obtain tissue for diagnosis is necessary when there is doubt about tumour type, and where the tumour's histological sub-type affects treatment and prognosis. For example, rhabdomyosarcoma, a tumour of 'embryonal' muscle, can occur in many sites in the body. It is necessary, therefore, to differentiate between this and other tumours that could occur in the same site so that the correct treatment may be given. Tissue obtained at operation for Wilms' tumour (nephroblastoma) is examined for histological type. 'Favourable' histology Wilms' tumour has a good prognosis and calls for less aggressive therapy than Wilms' of 'unfavourable' histology.

Specimens obtained at operation must be taken to histopathology as soon as possible. Special studies are performed on fresh tissue, rather than on tissue preserved in formalin.

It is possible to perform needle biopsies to obtain tissue samples from accessible sites, such as lymph nodes. 'Tru-cut' or needle biopsy spares the child, who may not be very fit, from a more hazardous operation. Many surgeons, however, prefer to carry out open biopsies to ensure a controlled procedure. This applies especially where there is a likelihood of bleeding, as in the liver, or of rupture of a contained tumour. In order to make a definite diagnosis the pathologist may require more tissue than a needle biopsy provides.

Treatment

Occasionally, before a treatment plan can begin, an emergency operation may be necessary to save the patient's life or to preserve neurological function. An emergency tracheostomy may be required to relieve airway obstruction due to nasopharyngeal, non-Hodgkin's lymphoma (NHL). Neuroblastoma arising from a paravertebral sympathetic ganglion can sometimes present with paraplegia. Decompression of the spinal cord is an urgent priority to prevent irreversible damage.

Recently, chemotherapy has been used in place of surgery as

a 'medical' laminectomy. Even with emergency treatment, return of function may be incomplete.

In the treatment of childhood malignancy today, surgery may be completely curative by primary excision of an encapsulated tumour, or it may be used in combination with chemotherapy and/or radiotherapy. Classifying a solid tumour as 'Stage I' indicates that it is contained and may be suitable for excision. Stage I Wilms' tumour is treated by nephrectomy followed by a short course of chemotherapy – treatment which is 95 per cent successful.

Tumours in which surgery can be completely curative include retinoblastoma, tumour of the eye, Stage I neuroblastoma, orchioblastoma, a tumour of the testis, and some brain tumours, such as cerebellar astrocytoma. Brain tumours that cannot be surgically removed because they are in, or adjacent to, vital structures, can be treated with radiotherapy, for example, brain stem gliomas.

Surgery is often delayed until after chemotherapy or radiotherapy has been used to reduce the size and spread of the tumour. Careful interdisciplinary discussion, with the help of modern imaging techniques, allows the team to choose the optimum time for the operation. This should lead to a reduction in the number of unnecessary initial operations. If excision of the tumour is incomplete, chemotherapy and/or radiotherapy is used to try to eradicate residual tumour. A 'second look' operation may then complete the removal process.

The present treatment for Stages III and IV neuroblastoma is a good example of the proper use of delayed surgery. The child receives four to eight months of chemotherapy prior to delayed excision of his primary neuroblastoma. The exact number of courses depends on the response of the tumour, measured by repeated investigations, such as CT scanning, as well as on the child's ability to recover from the toxic effects of the drugs.

Surgical removal of other tumours before chemotherapy and/or radiotherapy can result in unnecessary loss of function or removal of organs. Rhabdomyosarcoma of the bladder was once treated by complete pelvic exenteration. Amputation of limbs and other mutilating procedures may no longer be necessary to successfully treat the child with osteosarcoma or Ewing's sarcoma. It is possible for surgeons to carry out limb-preserving operations, in suitable cases, after treatment with chemotherapy and radiotherapy.

The most common site for metastases in paediatric solid tumours is the lung. Treatment of metastatic disease in the lung, liver and even occasionally the brain sometimes includes surgical removal, provided the primary disease is well controlled.

It takes time for clinical trials to indicate which combinations of therapy are most successful. Protocols continue to change in the light of these trials. Table 7.1 gives some indication of the place of surgery in the treatment of the more common types of childhood tumour.

Table 7.1   Potentially curative treatment modalities in childhood cancer

	Surgery	Radiotherapy	Chemotherapy
Hepatoblastoma	+	−	(+)
Neuroblastoma	+	−	+
Retinoblastoma	+	(+)	−
Non-Hodgkin's lymphoma	(+)	−	+
Acute lymphoblastic leukaemia	−	+	+
Hodgkin's disease	−	(+)	+
Ewing's sarcoma	(+)	+	+
Osteosarcoma	+	−	+
Brain tumours	+	+	(+)
Rhabdomyosarcoma	(+)	+	+
Wilms' tumour	+	(+)	+
Germ cell tumours	(+)	−	+

(+) indicates that the use of the modality may depend on stage of disease.
− may mean that the tumour is not suitable for that form of treatment, or that it is not used because of the extreme sensitivity of the tumour to chemotherapy.

Relief of Symptoms and Complications

At any time during the course of disease and treatment, surgery may be required to relieve symptoms or treat complications. Surgical emergencies related to treatment are not common but occasionally gut perforation or intussusception of tumour can occur. Symptoms related to raised intracranial pressure or obstructed cerebrospinal fluid flow, associated with some brain tumours, will need surgical shunting.

Patients with advanced disease in whom pain control is difficult may require operative measures, such as chordotomy, to relieve their distress.

Vascular and Cerebrospinal Fluid (CSF) Access

Last but not at all the least of the surgeon's contribution is the siting of indwelling intravenous and CSF access. All children requiring intensive regimes of chemotherapy will need good venous access; this is provided by the insertion under general anaesthetic of various types of indwelling catheters.

In rare circumstances a child may need frequent lumbar punctures for the administration of intrathecal drugs. To spare him the trauma of repeated procedures an intra-ventricular reservoir may be implanted by the neurosurgeon. These reservoirs also allow for better circulation of the cytotoxic drugs around the meninges. Very rarely, shunts may be needed to drain cerebrospinal or ascitic fluid.

The exact contribution of surgery in the management of a particular child will differ. Therefore, the nurse needs a good understanding of the overall treatment plan. Such understanding will help her to prepare and support the child and his family in the time available before the operation takes place.

SURGICAL NURSING

For some children with malignant disease, surgery will be the first step in treatment. Others will have already received chemotherapy or radiotherapy in the oncology unit.

In either circumstance, the time of surgery will be an extremely anxious one for the child and his family. They suffer the emotional strain that accompanies any operation. Added to that is the frightening question of what will be found at operation. Waiting three or more days for histology reports and answers to that question must be unbearably difficult. It is impossible to put oneself in the position of these parents watching a loved child suffering and having no power to heal all his emotional and physical pain.

Children having tumour excisions are usually admitted to a paediatric surgical unit. Most will require intensive nursing care postoperatively.

This change to new surroundings and unfamiliar staff at such a stressful time needs to be carefully managed. Ideally, the family's primary nurse from the oncology unit would continue to care for the child before and after surgery.

Nursing and medical staff on surgical wards can feel stressed by the presence of oncology patients. There seem to be several reasons for this. Despite preoperative visits and introductions, many staff feel they do not know the parents and child well enough to provide the close support that they need. Secondly – and this may be because of the types of patient they see – surgical nurses may have a more negative outlook towards the outcomes of oncology treatment.

The nature of surgical nursing, which has tight time-schedules and seems more orderly than oncology nursing, can lead to conflict between nurses' and parents' roles. Parents who have become experts in their child's condition, and have been involved in all nursing care on the oncology unit, may suddenly be thrown back to early feelings of uncertainty and fear by the new surroundings and the prospect of surgery. However, paediatric nurses in any speciality who practise family-centred nursing will all have the same goals. The focus of their care will be the whole child and nursing will be carried out in partnership with the parents. This philosophy of care is the basis of the following discussion about nursing the surgical oncology patient.

Preoperative Assessment

Before a plan of care can be discussed, the nurse needs to assess tactfully both the parents' and the child's understanding of the forthcoming surgery (Figure 7.2). Do they know the purpose of the surgery? Are their expectations of postoperative progress realistic? How much have they been told about preoperative preparation and anaesthesia? To assess their reactions and feelings it is important to talk about previous hospital experiences. Has any family member had surgery before? How did that affect them? Has their past experience of hospitals been good or otherwise? How have they coped with blood tests, intravenous therapy and oncology treatment?

Psychological – understanding, coping
Social – home routines, family care
Physical – nutrition, circulation, infection
Family – understanding, ability to assist with care
Medical – reason for surgery, type of procedures, previous therapy

Figure 7.2   Preoperative assessment

This is an important time for creating a friendly, supportive atmosphere which the family will need in the days to come.

Accurate information given in a confident, organised manner will help build trust. Research evidence indicates that ignorance produces fear but that sufficient information helps people to cope (La Montagne, 1987). Time must be taken to get close to the child and his family, perhaps during orientation to the unit, or over coffee in the ward during a quiet evening spell. If the family can feel comfortable with their nurse they will be better able to express their deep concerns about the surgery.

Are they ignoring potential outcomes completely? How do they feel about what is to happen – about imminent changes in appearance or body function? Is the child reacting appropriately? And what do they feel is the best way for their child to be prepared psychologically for his operation?

In order to assist the parents to provide a secure environment for their child in hospital, the nurse must discover what their routines are at home.

As far as possible nursing care should be planned around usual family care. After the operation a swift return to these routines will help the child's return to normality.

Specific points should be noted in the physical assessment. There may be evidence of disease-related symptoms such as pain, altered mobility, anaemia or bleeding. Previous treatment with chemotherapy or radiotherapy may have left the child in a poor nutritional state. A period of intravenous feeding will sometimes be prescribed to improve his chances of full recovery from surgery. Measurement of temperature and examination of skin and mouth could indicate the presence of infection requiring antibiotic treatment.

Obviously the child's general condition will affect his recovery from major surgery, but there is no evidence to suggest that adjuvant chemotherapy delays wound healing. Radiotherapy is not usually commenced until 10–14 days after surgery and wound healing should be complete in that time. Previous radiotherapy to the operative area, however, can result in problems with adhesions as well as slower healing.

To complete the admission assessment, the nurse should record the extent to which parents wish to be involved in the care of their child. Are they resident for the duration of his stay? Do they want to be present for all procedures? What further teaching and support do they need to assist with nursing care? Have they made suitable provision for siblings? Are there any other problems which could be sorted out now to prevent outside worries adding to their stress at a crucial time?

Preoperative Care Planning

Preparation for operation will depend on the nature of the surgery, as well as on the findings of the assessment. Specific problems which need preoperative consideration relate to the tumour type. For example, catecholamine release in patients with neuroblastoma may cause severe hypertension. Blood pressure monitoring and control with medication will be necessary before operation.

The child who must undergo an amputation for osteosarcoma will need help to work through his anticipatory grieving. He and his family must have expert counselling to support them in dealing with their anger and depression. Nursing staff, while coping with their own emotional response to such an event, should understand the natural reactions of the child and his parents to this traumatic occurrence. The advice and support of a specialist social worker or psychologist should be sought.

The most important aim of preoperative care is to ensure understanding so as to minimise fear.

Age-appropriate explanations by nurse or parent should be given in reasonable time to help adjustment to places and events. Play can be used to introduce new equipment, to illustrate explanations and to assist expression of feelings.

Anxiety at such time is a completely normal reaction – it would be worrying to find no anxiety in the family. The purpose of nursing interventions related to anxiety is to keep the anxiety at a manageable level. The parents will cease to be effective and the child will suffer unnecessarily if the degree of stress is too great.

Evaluation of Care

To discover whether the measures taken have achieved the stated goals the nurse can first ask the parents if they feel the child is behaving appropriately. Is he withdrawn, aggressive, unnaturally cheerful? Is he sleeping badly, crying easily, ignoring them? By observing his interaction with others and his play, the nurse may identify particular things that are worrying him.

The child's and parents' understanding of events can be reassessed by asking them to repeat explanations or to describe events in their own words.

Observation of physical signs will indicate any abnormality necessitating changes in care, or even postponement of surgery.

Recording of normal parameters in the preoperative period is important for comparison with observations made during and after surgery.

Intraoperative Care

The findings made during surgery will affect the duration of the procedure. Thus it is impossible to give parents and relatives an accurate estimate of how long it will be before their child returns to the ward – a major excision could take as long as eight hours. They will need to fill this time somehow. If the parents can be persuaded to go out for a walk, go home for a few hours, have a bath, they will manage the waiting better than if they sit beside an empty bed throughout.

Sometimes staff receive progress reports which could be passed on to the parents in a suitably comforting manner.

In the time available the nurse and parents can draw up the postoperative care plan. Besides occupying and involving the parents, this serves as a further teaching session about what to expect on their child's return. Parents must be encouraged to take regular short breaks from the intensive area so that they can remain effective for their child. Discussing, in advance, the arrangements for parents to relieve each other will ensure less resistance to the idea when the time comes.

Postoperative Assessment, Care and Evaluation

Nursing assessment and care of the paediatric oncology patient in the immediate postoperative period is essentially the same as for any child undergoing similar surgery. Physiological condition and function is the first concern as the nurse assesses breathing, circulation, hydration, output, the surgical wound and the child's need for pain relief.

The body responds to major surgery and removal of tissue by retaining water and sodium, so the child's fluid input must be restricted for the first few days. Monitoring of central venous pressure and arterial pressures is usually necessary, as is careful measurement of output and body weight. Regular estimations of serum electrolytes and blood sugar allow corrective treatment to be prescribed.

Pain can be assessed even in the unconscious child by observation of pulse and blood pressure, of facial expression, body posture and muscle tension.

Once the child's condition is stable, attention can be focused

Figure 7·3 An example of a postoperative care plan

Identified need	Goal	Nursing intervention	Child's self-care	Care by parent
Safe recovery from anaesthetic	Child will maintain normal respiration	Provide oxygen and suction for emergency use. Nurse in recovery position; sit up when conscious to enable chest expansion. Observe colour and respirations	Deep breathing and try to cough	Assist with positioning. Every 2 hours encourage deep breathing and coughing
Comfort	Child will be pain-free and comfortable; will be able to express anxiety	Assess pain. Administer analgesia as required. Explain events and give comfort to child and parent	Complain if anywhere hurts	Give comfort. Encourage expression of fears
Restricted fluids	Child will be prevented from becoming fluid overloaded	Administer i.v. fluids as prescribed. Hourly fluid balance totals. Weigh 12-hourly		Continue Broviac catheter care and dressing. Assist with weighing

Identified need	Goal	Nursing intervention	Child's self-care	Care by parent
Safe recovery from surgery	Child will not develop an infection, haemorrhage, or have other complications	Observe temperature, pulse, BP, CVP. Check wound and assess drainage. Test all urine with 6-hourly Dextrostix	To understand (age-appropriate) reasons for care	Keep wound area clean and dry. Try to prevent tension on wound when moving child
	Child will have swift return of normal gut function	Aspirate NG tube. Check bowel sounds. Record bowel function. Re-introduce fluid and diet when appropriate	Nothing to eat or drink until he is able	Remind about nil-by-mouth. Assist with drink and food when these are allowed
Assistance with activities of living	Child's activities of living will be as near normal as possible	Assist mother	As soon as able child can clean teeth, wash and dress, walk to toilet	Give mouthcare 2-hourly until drinking. Attend to child's toilet and hygiene needs.
		Encourage gradual mobilisation		Encourage child to move about and to care for himself. Involve child in play activities

on comfort, mobility and hygiene needs. When conscious he may express fear related to pain, uncertainty or disorientation. The presence of his parents and familiar sights and sounds will quickly dispel uncertainty – as will age-appropriate explanations of events and surroundings. Pain must be controlled with adequate analgesia.

The care plan (Figure 7.3) is an example of care for a child who has had a laparotomy and excision of abdominal neuro-blastoma. As is common in paediatric surgery, the sutures are subcuticular and there is no wound dressing. Evaluation of care again takes the form of observation and reassessment. Has the analgesia removed or reduced pain-related symptoms? Is the child's weight static over twenty-four hours? Is his mouth clean and moist?

The effectiveness of supportive measures is extremely difficult to assess as so many factors are involved. What do we mean by support? If the child appears to adapt well to altered body function or the loss of a limb, who can say which particular nursing action contributed to his adaptation?

Information aids coping, so helping the family to understand something will reduce their anxiety. But the effect of measures aimed at providing emotional comfort can only be guessed at. It is unlikely that any family would ever approach surgical treatment with joy. However, if they feel welcome, at ease with staff and able to talk, then supportive measures are probably working.

CONCLUSION

There is no doubt that surgery, as part of the management of childhood cancer, is a stressful event. Whether the surgical procedure is diagnostic, therapeutic or for other reasons, the child and his family need care and support as well as accurate information. The nurse, as a member of the oncology team, can best meet these needs by using a family-centred approach.

Today, the treatment of malignant disease in children is frequently successful. As a result the long-term effects of therapy are now becoming evident. Each child will react in a different way to the experience of having an operation. Whether the child is cured or not, nursing and family care can help him to recover from his surgery.

Reference

La Montagne L (1987) Children's pre-operative coping: replication and extension. *Nursing Research*, **36**(3): 163-167.

Further Reading

Hayes D (ed.) (1986) *Paediatric Surgical Oncology*. Orlando: Grune and Stratton.

McClanahan M (1984) Surgery. In: *Complete Guide to Cancer Nursing*, Beyers M, Werner J and Durbury S (eds.), pp. 68-132. London: Edward Arnold.

Plaschkes J (1986) Surgical oncology in children. In: *Cancer in Children. Clinical Management*, 2nd edn. Voute P, Barrett A, Bloom H, Lemerle J and Neidhardt M (eds.), pp. 46-53. Berlin: Springer-Verlag.

Whaley L and Wong D (1987) *Nursing Care of Infants and Children*, St Louis: C V Mosby.

8
The Child and Bone Marrow Transplantation

BONE MARROW TRANSPLANTATION

Bone marrow transplantation (BMT) has become an accepted treatment for leukaemia and some forms of solid tumours, for example, lymphomas, aplastic anaemia and severe forms of combined immune deficiency syndromes. Since 1970, over 6,000 individuals worldwide have received BMT for acute leukaemia. The choice for offering a child BMT depends on the prognostic factors of the child's disease.

Acute myeloid leukaemia (AML) is rare in children, accounting for only one-fifth of childhood leukaemia. Remission rates have improved with chemotherapy. However, over the last fifteen years BMT has emerged as the preferred treatment for AML in first remission.

The classification of acute lymphoblastic leukaemia (ALL) prognostic factors, i.e. clinical and laboratory features at presentation which predict the length of anticipated remission, has improved from simple findings such as age and presenting white blood counts to a series of involved scoring systems which include morphological, immunological and sometimes cytogenic findings. The aim of this is to define children of high risk of relapse who may benefit from the more intensive treatments such as BMT. However, even in the most intricate scoring systems the presenting white blood count remains the most reliable determinant of prognosis. Children who present with a high white blood cell count who have T cell disease or who have relapsed on completing conventional ALL treatment are given the option of BMT if a donor is available.

Chronic granulocytic leukaemia (CGL) accounts for less than 5 per cent of childhood leukaemia. Long-term survival rates with chemotherapy alone is nil. BMT is now the treatment of choice for childhood CGL.

Currently there are three types of transplant available:

- from a human leucocyte antigen (HLA) identical sibling;
- from a partial or fully HLA matched related or unrelated donor (these types of transplants are known as allogenic); and
- autologous transplantation. This is where the child's own bone marrow is harvested when in remission and cryo-preserved for reinfusion at a later date.

Tissue Typing

Prior to any definite plans about which type of BMT is to be carried out, the first step must be to tissue-type the child and his family, to determine whether there is a match-related donor. As each individual has a specific blood type determined by antigens present on the red blood cells, each individual also has a specific tissue type determined by four antigens which are present on white blood cells and fixed tissue. Human leucocyte antigen (HLA) is the name given to the antigen complex carried on chromosome 6, which determines the tissue type. A child will inherit two antigens from each of its parents. Therefore a parent usually only has two antigens the same as each of their children and would only be able to be used as a mismatched donor. The chance of siblings inheriting the same two antigens is 1 in 4. Therefore sibling donors are the most common. An identical twin is the ideal donor.

Another test of histocompatibility is mixed lymphocyte culture (MLC). T lymphocytes which mediate tissue rejection from the child and the potential donor are cultured together. If there is no reactivity after seven days this shows compatibility and confirms the compatibility of the HLA-matched donor. If a child does not have any siblings, it is possible to attempt to find a matched, unrelated donor (MUD) by submitting the child's tissue typing to the Anthony Nolan Tissue Bank.

Pre-transplantation Work-up

Once tissue-typing information has been confirmed and the type of transplant decided upon, the child – if old enough to understand the explanation – his parents and possibly other members of the immediate family are seen by the medical staff and the child's primary nurse. The procedure of transplantation is explained fully. An explanation of why BMT is the treatment of choice should be given. The family are asked not to give their immediate response but are given the opportunity to discuss whether or not to accept transplant. In practice, very few reject the offer. When transplantation has been accepted, a programme of events should be formulated. A copy of this should be given to the parents and, if appropriate, the child, so that they are aware of what is to happen and when. This allows for forward planning of family life.

Good health is of paramount importance. The child should be in a good nutritional state. Weight loss associated with previous chemotherapy should be replaced. Referral to the nurse nutritionist should be of value as advice pre-, during and post-transplant can be given on dietary needs and supplements. The disease status must be reassessed, the child should be in bone marrow remission and have no evidence of leukaemic deposits in the central nervous system, skin or testes. Full infection screening should be carried out, including assessment of cytomegalovirus status (CMV). If the child is CMV negative all subsequent transfusions of blood and platelets should be CMV negative. A full dental examination should be performed and any dental caries dealt with. Routine chest X-ray, electro-cardiogram (ECG), haematological status, chemical pathology, liver function and clotting screen are undertaken. Glomerular filtration rate is estimated to ensure there is no renal impairment prior to the giving of high dose chemotherapy. Central venous access is essential. A Hickman right atrial catheter is inserted under general anaesthesia one week prior to transplantation, to allow time for healing. A Hickman catheter allows safe, intravenous entry and removes the distressing need for multiple venepunctures over the possible four to six weeks of hospital-isation and regular outpatient appointments over the following months.

The family should be introduced to the other members of the ward team including the play therapist who will enter the isolation cubicle and provide appropriate play or diversional therapy for the child and give parents a well-earned and often needed break. The social worker will make contact with the family so that any financial or social problems can be discussed.

Education is often a great worry to the parents and adolescents approaching examinations. Home tuition should be arranged for the first six months post-BMT for any child of school age.

Total body irradiation (TBI) is a component of the cyto-reduction programme. It is necessary to perform test doses prior to the day of TBI to measure and record the dose variation of the child's skull, upper lung, lower lung, and abdomen in both positions adopted for treatment – supine and lateral. Semi-conduct probes are placed over these sites for two minutes. From these measurements the treatment time required for each individual child will be calculated. This gives the parents and an older child the opportunity to discuss with the radiotherapist the method of treatment, and to familiarise the child with the treatment room. Many younger children return from the TBI unit explaining that they have been in a big space ship.

Sedation is very rarely needed for children over the age of three for the test doses. But all patients are sedated on the day of TBI. Oral cyclosporine A (CSA), 8 mg/kg/day, in two divided doses, is started at seven days before allografting in order to prevent graft versus host disease (GVH). Ingenuity is needed by the parents to disguise this very unpalatable substance which must be taken six months post-transplant. CSA is not required for autografting, as there will be no graft versus host disease (GVH).

Admission

Admission should occur the day prior to cyto-reduction commencing. This allows time for the child, his parents and siblings to familiarise themselves with their environment. Personal belongings, such as the child's own clothes, favourite toys, videos and computers should be brought in with them. Decoration by the child and his parents of the cubicle should be encouraged, enabling the child to personalise the room which is going to be his living room, playroom and bedroom for the next few weeks. Parents must be given the opportunity to stay with their child. A bed should be provided for the parent who wishes to sleep in the cubicle. Cooking and laundry facilities should be made available.

Base-line observations of temperature, pulse, respiration rate, blood pressure, urine analysis, height and weight should be noted. A full nursing history will establish the child's normal sleeping pattern, educational status, relationships with his peer group, food likes and dislikes. It is very important to determine the child's understanding of his illness. This can be achieved by talking to the child, or with the older child or adolescent asking them to write down in their own words their knowledge of the illness. This should be included in the care plan. It is often valuable to talk to an adolescent when his parents are not present. Many will feel inhibited by their parents and protective towards them, sometimes not wishing to express their fears because they may upset mum and dad.

Care of the Bone Marrow Donor

The sibling who is to donate marrow must undertake a full medical examination prior to the finalisation of the transplant programme. The examination should include chest X-ray, ECG, blood chemistry and a full haematological screen, to ensure they are fit for general anaesthesia. If the child is old enough he should donate one unit of blood, so that it may be used post-harvest as an autologous transfusion. Parents should be given this option to reduce any anxiety which may be associated with donor transfusion. Explanation of the procedure should be given to the child at a level he will understand.

The donor is admitted prior to the recipient receiving TBI or if the child is to have chemotherapy alone prior to this being given. It should be suggested to the parents that if possible both of them or another relative/friend should also be present in the hospital, so that they do not feel torn between their ill child and the donor. The donor has bone marrow removed under general anaesthesia. The site of choice for bone marrow aspiration is the posterior iliac crest, but the anterior iliac crest and the sternum may be used.

Bone marrow harvesting is the procedure to extract viable stem cells. Stem cells are haemopoetic cells that are capable of replication and differentiation into the major blood cell lines. (The number of cells required for haemopoetic reconstitution is one times ten to the ten nucleative marrow cells.) In the theatre the marrow is processed into a single cell suspension for infusion. The volume harvested is replaced by the blood transfusion and intravenous fluids are given until the child is awake and able to take oral fluids. At the end of the harvest, pressure dressings are applied to the puncture sites. The postoperative period is usually free from complications although soreness at the site is common. On discharge the following day, the child is given iron tablets and folic acid to be taken for two weeks. Harvesting from the donor is timed to coincide with the completion of the preparation of the recipient.

Autologous bone marrow harvesting follows the same procedure as that for allogenic transplantation with the exception of the processing which can allow for long periods of time until the bone marrow is used. The reinfusion can take place on the

Figure 8.1 Nursing care plan 1 – High-dose chemotherapy

Problem/Need	Goal	Nursing action
Potential side-effects of high-dose chemotherapy. Nausea, vomiting, electrolyte and fluid imbalance, renal impairment	To prevent excess nausea and vomiting. To prevent fluid overload; to prevent renal impairment. To detect electrolyte imbalance early. Child and parent to comprehend need for actions to be taken following administration of therapy	1. Check renal function is adequate prior to administration of chemotherapy 2. Administer chemotherapy regime as prescribed 3. Strict recording of fluid balance intake and output. Nappies of young children to be weighed. Child to be encouraged to void urine regularly 4. Observe for signs of overload – oedema, breathlessness, rising blood pressure. 5. Diuretics to be given as required to maintain fluid balance 6. Hourly recordings of blood pressure, pulse, respiration during intensive hydration. Four hourly thereafter 7. Weight measured daily or more frequently if imbalance suspected 8. Observe urinary status and test daily 9. Anti-emetics to be given regularly, and effectiveness to be monitored 10. Daily monitoring of urea and electolytes. If imbalance occurs more frequent sampling may be necessary 11. Full explanation to be given to the child and his parents of actions being taken. Parents to be involved in care

day of the harvest or years later. The stem cells are protected with diamethylsulphoxide (DMSO) which protects the bone marrow from lysis during freezing. The marrow is stored in liquid nitrogen until the patient requires it.

Preparation of the Recipient

To achieve profound immunosuppression and increase leukaemic cell kill, a combination of high-dose chemotherapy and TBI is given prior to BMT (see Figures 8.1 and 8.3).

Total Body Irradiation

TBI is given to eradicate the child's own bone marrow so destroying his immunity and destroying any outstanding leukaemic cells in sanctuary sites. TBI lasts for about 280 minutes, during which time the child has to lie very still (Figure 8.2). The position is changed from supine to lateral, at which time, if the child wishes, he can stretch and move around slightly. About three hours after TBI starts sickness may become a problem. This only occurs in about 40 per cent of the children. They are rarely warned by a feeling of nausea. To try to prevent this a premedication of oral phenobarbitone and dexamethasone is given the evening prior to TBI and again intravenously on the morning of the procedure. This helps to prevent radiation induced cerebral oedema and associated nausea. Further sedation can be given so that the child is sleepy and not distressed. This may need to be repeated at regular intervals.

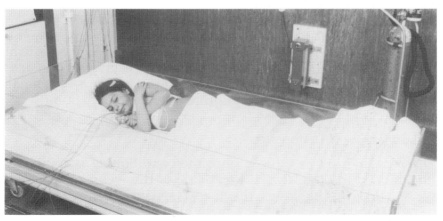

Figure 8.2   Child in position for total body irradiation in the TBI unit

A young child should be transferred to the TBI unit dressed in his own pyjamas, accompanied by his favourite teddy, toy or comfort blanket. Many parents carry their small children. The child is made comfortable in the unit and the parents leave. A second nurse should accompany the parents back to the ward. Many say that this is the time they fear the most. There is no turning back once TBI has been given. They feel lonely and isolated. This day seems the longest day of their lives. The child's favourite cassettes can be played to him by means of a radio-link, and the patient is constantly observed using closed circuit television. A two-way microphone is in the room, so communication can be maintained throughout. Intravenous fluids are maintained and regular sedation given. If the child becomes distressed, wants to vomit or micturate or needs a cuddle, the radiation can be switched off and the nurse may go in. On completion of the TBI the child is returned to the ward. Parotitis may occur within twelve hours of TBI, but resolves within 48 hours. Regular analgesia may be required for earache. Other immediate side-effects are a dry mouth – artificial saliva is of value in such cases. Transient erythema may be present for about 24 hours. Nausea, vomiting and diarrhoea last for varying periods of time and will need controlling with anti-emetic and anti-diarrhoeal agents. Pyrexia may follow TBI. This usually passes within 12 hours. Anti-pyretic agents should be given.

Intermediate side-effects are alopecia, two weeks onwards; pneumonitis may manifest two or three weeks after treatment; somnolence usually presents four to six weeks later, and if the child is at home he may need re-admitting for intravenous fluids if oral intake is compromised by prolonged periods of sleep.

Late side-effects of TBI include cataracts in about 20 per cent of the children at four years, sterility and growth impairment. The children who receive TBI should be monitored regularly at growth clinics. Growth hormones should be given if needed. Parents are taught to administer the injections. In a very small percentage of patients a second primary growth may occur.

Bone Marrow Infusion

The bone marrow is infused once the conditioning is complete. It is infused through the Hickman line of the recipient, where it passes first to the lungs, liver and spleen, then after 10–20 days it can be detected in the bone marrow. Many parents find the transplant itself an anti-climax after the intensive programme of the cytoreduction, or become rather euphoric during it, as it signals the start of the cure.

Post-Transplant Care

There now follows the most hazardous period for the child, where good reverse barrier nursing plays a vital part in his survival. He will for nearly two weeks have no neutrophils and virtually no platelets, so rendering him prone to overwhelming infection and haemorrhage. Although it is stressed to the parents and children that a protected environment is essential to the success of the transplant, the effect of the isolation may be very severe on both the child and his parents. The nurse should be sensitive to this and aware of the possibility of changes of behaviour. Adolescents often find it difficult to deal with isolation and conflict commonly arises within the family group. The adolescent finds it difficult to accept temporary, complete dependence on his parents, nursing and medical staff. Regression to a more childish role can occur in attempts to gain security and parental support. Parents and children often show great ingenuity in personalising their rooms to allow for many activities. Parents should be encouraged to cook, launder clothes and practise a home routine as much as possible.

The needs of the siblings should not be forgotten. The play therapist is invaluable in maintaining this link and in devising games that can be played through a door. The constraints of isolation on a young child where a parent or grandparent stays with him have been found not to be unduly stressful. Involvement of parents in the child's care is essential. Early detection of infection is vital. Regular four-hourly temperature, pulse, respiration rate and blood pressure are of paramount importance in detecting early signs of infection, notably septicaemia. Any pyrexia of 38°C or above, rising pulse rate or a falling blood pressure should be reported immediately. Full infection screening should be performed, and the child commence an intravenous, broad spectrum antibiotic. Vigilance must still be maintained for signs of improvement or deterioration on this regime. Furthermore, specific antibiotics or systematic *Candida* treatment may be required. Failure to diagnose infection early in these children can lead to a rapid death. Infection is most likely to be caused by the child's own body flora gram negative rods. This must be stressed to the parents because many feel that it was a shortcoming in their nursing technique which gave the child an infection.

Figure 8.3 Nursing care plan 2 – Total body irradiation

Problem/Need	Goal	Nursing action
Potential infection due to low white cell count secondary to high dose chemotherapy and TBI	To detect infection and treat early, to prevent further deterioration.	1. Four-hourly temperature, pulse, blood pressure and respiration rates to be recorded
	To relieve symptoms and keep the child comfortable while infection is present.	2. Full infection screening, including taking blood cultures if temperature above 38°C
	To ensure parents are aware of the need for early detection and enable them to report suspected change in their child's condition	3. Repeat culture if temperature remains elevated. Always repeat culture prior to any change in antibiotics
		4. Encourage high oral fluid intake while pyrexial. Intravenous supplementation may be necessary
		5. Give antipyretic agents
		6. Nurse the child with a safe fan in situ. Tepid sponge child if he will tolerate this – usually tolerated better when performed by the mother
		7. Observe for any adverse reactions to antibiotics, i.e. diarrhoea, rashes
		8. Full explanation to parents
		9. Appropriate explanation to child (age-related)

Mouth care with oral anti-fungal preparations and frequent oral inspection are essential. Oral candidiasis often occurs. Oral fungal infection can rapidly lead to oesophageal candidiasis and even to *Candida pneumonia*. Encouragement is not enough, as not all children will carry out mouth care efficiently, particularly when their mouths are sore. Many parents perform the care for their children, but some feel that this is too distressing, particularly when the child is ill and the mouth sore. The nurse must then step in and often act as the 'not quite so kind' person, leaving mum to give the cuddles and rewards. Adequate analgesia in the form of a continual diamorphine infusion is essential, because *Candida* is often secondary to severe mucositis associated with high-dose chemotherapy. Parents should be taught to be vigilant in recognising signs of infection or bleeding, as they usually attend to the child's toilet and hygiene needs. A daily full wash is needed to reduce skin flora.

Susceptibility to infection is prolonged, due to immunosuppression; and partly due to the use of the drug Cyclosporine A which is given to allograft patients to prevent GVH. Cyclosporine inhibits the production of T lymphocytes in the graft, which would stimulate the immune system to reject the host as foreign and antibody production by B lymphocytes is depressed. Early recognition of GVH disease is essential. The organs which can be affected are the skin, gastrointestinal tract and liver. GVH disease can vary in degree from transient to moderate to severe forms. It is, however, proof that engraftment has taken place.

GVH disease of the skin grades I and II consist of a maculopapular rash on the palms and soles, and often in children on the cheeks. This may be transient and respond to intravenous high-dose methylprednisolone. Grades III and IV GVH present as red raw blisters which resemble burns. The junction of the epidermis and dermis may separate, leaving large, raw areas prone to secondary infection. The child with mild skin GVH disease is hypersensitive to extremes of temperature. As the condition becomes more severe pain becomes a problem. The skin cannot be touched and intravenous diamorphine by means of a continuous infusion should be given. The child should be nursed as one would nurse a major burns case. Dehydration, fluid loss and electrolyte imbalance are major problems, requiring frequent monitoring and correction. The child should be nursed on a foam sponge to help the absorption of serous fluid, thereby relieving the possibility of secondary infection.

Figure 8.4 Nursing care plan 3 – GVH disease of the gut

Problem/Need	Goal	Nursing action
Potential GVH disease of gut. Abdominal pain, diarrhoea	To detect GVH disease early. To eliminate GVH disease of gut. To relieve abdominal pain. To reduce diarrhoea. To control diarrhoea. To detect early signs of gastro-intestinal bleeding. Parents and child to be fully informed of potential problems	1. Keep child's buttocks as clean as possible and free from soreness. Apply barrier cream where ever necessary
		2. Give adequate analgesia and anti-diarrhoeal agent. Support patient and parents through the child's bouts of severe abdominal pain
		3. Inspection of stools: amount, colour, consistency, presence of blood, mucous, tissue and Cyclosporine A
		4. Record biochemistry levels and fluid balance
		5. Prevention of infection around anal area by careful cleansing
		6. Careful handling of stool specimens
		7. Collect stool specimens twice daily

The raw, wet or infected areas should be covered with Flamazine cream, the dry areas with white, soft paraffin to rehydrate the skin from outside in. If the GVH disease extends to the eyes they are treated with steroid eye drops. Constant reassurance must be given to the child and parents that even this severe form of GVH disease is capable of healing with the skin returning to normal and no further eruptions seen. It can, however, become a chronic skin condition.

GVH disease of the gut usually presents with abdominal pain, cramp and diarrhoea which resembles mincemeat. This may be transient, lasting only a few days and fluid loss is minimal. If uncontrolled or unresponsive to steroids litres of fluid may be passed as diarrhoea in 24 hours. The stools should be observed for the presence of Cyclosporine A. This makes the stools appear oily. If present it may be necessary to administer CSA intravenously (see Figure 8.4).

GVH Disease of the Liver

GVH disease of the liver usually presents with abnormal liver function tests, jaundice of the sclera and skin, clotting abnormalities, pruritic rash, and the stools may be bulky and pale. The picture can be from mild jaundice with a cholestatic picture to complete liver failure (see Figure 8.5).

Chronic GVH disease can appear after 70 days when there has been no acute GVH disease. The same organs are usually involved. The chronic form of skin GVH disease is often scar-like eruptions which look like lichen. Chronic liver disease resembles primary biliary cirrhosis. When the gut is involved malabsorption develops with or without chronic diarrhoea.

Acute GVH disease is present in about 70 per cent of patients given a graft. Chronic GVH disease happens in about 25 per cent of long-term survivors. In many cases the GVH disease is transient, but the severe GVH disease still accounts for much of the mortality and morbidity of transplant patients. Very occasionally, the graft may not take. This is a devastating experience for all. Intense support must be given to the child and parents. Without engraftment of donor marrow there is no hope of survival. The child will have to be reconditioned and the whole process repeated.

Figure 8.5   Nursing care plan 4 – GVH disease of the liver

Problem/Need	Goal	Nursing action
Potential GVH disease of the liver	To detect GVH disease early To eliminate GVH disease of the liver. To maintain normal clotting factors. To alleviate any distressing and unpleasant side-effects. To have a well-informed, well-supported family and patient	1. Monitor liver function and clotting factors daily. 2. Observe patient for any obvious signs of jaundice 3. Give antihistamine if rash is apparent and distressing 4. Observe stools for signs of obstructive jaundice 5. Test urine for urobilinogen 6. Observe for fitting or twitching if bilirubin is high 7. Keep parents fully in the picture. Answer questions honestly. Support if condition appears to be deteriorating further

Powles Syndrome

This is pulmonary oedema with leaky endothelial system syndrome, devastating complication of transplant, particularly mismatch. Its presentation follows five to ten days after transplant. The patient's temperature rises, weight increases, central venous pressure (CVP) is negative, serum albumen is low and the child is in a positive fluid balance. What has occurred is that fluid has entered the extra cellular spaces because of the low serum albumen. Intravenous albumen should be given and the CVP checked. When it begins to rise the child should be given diuretics. This can be repeated to maintain a negative fluid balance. If this does not work and serum albumen and CVP continue to fall, it is symptomatic of crashing pulmonary oedema. The blood gases will deteriorate within a very short space of time as the lungs fill with fluid because of the leaky endothelial system. The treatment for this is intermittent positive pressure ventilation. The alveoli become inelastic, damage occurs to vital organs and the child dies. This shows the need for a constantly accurate record of fluid balance and a high nurse–patient ratio to allow for very close monitoring of the child's condition from hour to hour.

Cyclosporine A (CSA) is a complicated structure of amino acids and is produced by the fungal species tolycladium inflalum. It prevents T lymphocyte response without any toxicity to the haemopoetic cells. Cyclosporine A does have toxic effects on other systems. Overdosage or combined toxicity with other nephrotoxic drugs causes acute renal failure, requiring dialysis. Recovery from this is usual but may require three weeks of haemodialysis. Convulsions appear to be more common in children taking CSA, so prophylactic phenytoin is given. Phenytoin levels must be taken to ensure that the therapeutic dose has been achieved.

Other side-effects that can be a problem for the patient include hirsutism. This is very common and can be very distressing. Scalp hair tends to grow very well but may be very curly and coarse. Tremor can be slight or severe and appetite may be suppressed. This can be a problem in young children. All these effects go when the drug is stopped.

Follow-up Post-Transplant

Discharge usually occurs twenty-one days post-transplant, if the child's haematological and physical state allows. If the family do not live within travelling distance of the unit, prior arrangements should be made either for follow-up at their local oncology centre or for temporary accommodation in the area. It is important that close observation of haematological, biochemical and physical condition is kept so that appropriate action may be taken. The child usually attends the outpatient department twice weekly initially, the time between visits lengthening as the child's condition improves. Discharge medication should include CSA, phenytoin and oral anti-fungal agents. The latter continue for as long as the child is immunosuppressed by taking CSA. Septrin is given as a prophylactic measure against Pneumocystis. Close monitoring of the blood picture is needed, as bone marrow suppression can occur. Norethisterone should be given to teenage girls. This is usually commenced pre-transplant and continued post-transplant until the platelet count is adequate to allow the normal menstrual cycle to recommence.

Maintenance chemotherapy may be given to children who have received autologous transplants. For the first six months after transplant the child is susceptible to infections so should avoid crowded places, including school, takeaway food or reheated food and people who have infections. If the child has a direct contact with chicken-pox or measles he must receive immunoglobulin. Despite these restrictions, the child and family should be encouraged to lead as normal a life as possible, maintaining a small circle of friends, eating a normal diet to replenish weight loss which will have occurred during transplant.

Throughout the child's stay in hospital, close links should be maintained with the child's referring hospital, health visitor, GP and social workers. Financial help may be needed for travelling expenses and if one parent has temporarily to leave work to care for a child who is unable to attend playschool or full-time education.

The older child or the parents of the young child should be taught how to care for the Hickman line and to inspect for signs of bleeding, infection, excessive weight loss, abnormal bowel actions or skin rashes, and given a contact number to ring if there are any problems.

Going from the relatively safe environment of an isolation room can reduce the hardiest of parents to over-emotional people doubting their own capabilities of caring for their child. It cannot be stressed enough to them that without their help, their twenty-four hour physical and psychological care, the child would not have coped with this form of treatment. Parents form an invaluable part of the caring team.

Further Reading

Artinian B M (1983) Fostering hope in the bone marrow child. *Maternal Child Nurse Journal*, **1:** 57-71.

Barrett A J and Gordon Smith E C (1983) *Bone Marrow Transplantation – A Review*. Sponsored by Sandoz Products Ltd, produced by Medical Educational Services Ltd.

Bater M (1987) *Leukaemia Unit, The Royal Marsden Hospital, Sutton*. Presented at Third Annual Meeting, European Bone Marrow Transplantation Group, Interlaken, 1–5 March.

Chessells J M (1987) Acute leukaemia in children. *Clinics in Haematology*, chapter 8, pp 11-20.

De Boer Els (1984) *Young Child in Isolation: 1–5 Years Old*. Leiden, Holland: Kinderklinik Isolatie, Academisch Ziekenhuis.

Edwards J (1984) Mismatch bone marrow transplant. *Nursing Mirror,* **159** (2): 31-32.

Gale R P (1977) *Bone marrow transplantation in acute leukaemia. Lancet,* **2:** 1197-1200.

Stream P (1983) *Functions of the Outpatient Clinic Before and After Transplantation*. Symposium on Bone Marrow Transplantation. *Nursing Clinics of North America,* **18**(3): 603-609.

Stream P, Harrington E and Clark M (1980). Bone marrow transplantation, an option for children with acute leukaemia. *Cancer Nursing,* **3**(3): 195-199.

9

The Adolescent with Cancer

INTRODUCTION

Cohen and Wellisch (1978) report that the experience of cancer patients and their families has been described as 'living in limbo'. As survival time has lengthened for children with cancer, few studies have paid special attention to the unique difficulties experienced by the adolescent patient and his family. Improved prognosis means that the adolescent and his family have to cope with long-term uncertainty but, in many cases, with a realistic hope for cure. Improved survival among adolescents with cancer as with young children results from advances in chemotherapy, radiotherapy and surgery. It is true to say that cancer in the adolescent population can now be viewed as with other age groups as a chronic disease.

The types of cancer common in the adolescent age group are the acute leukaemias, lymphomas – Hodgkin's and non-Hodgkin's – central nervous system tumours and bone tumours such as osteogenic sarcoma and Ewing's sarcoma. As with younger children, it must be remembered that cancer in adolescence is rare yet accounts for significant morbidity and mortality.

Klopovich and Clancy (1985) describe the period of adolescence as a difficult time even under the best circumstances. Concerns of maturity, independence and sexual identity are tasks faced. When an adolescent develops a chronic, life-threatening disease, the entire emotional atmosphere surrounding him changes. Too often parents, family, physician and nurse become so concerned about the disease process that they overlook and, indeed in some instances, do not comprehend the feelings and concern the young person has about himself. Health care professionals must recognise and understand that adolescents with cancer are normal human beings at a special time in their lives, faced with the additional stress of a diagnosis of cancer. To care for the adolescent with cancer effectively, health professionals must have knowledge about growth and development specific to this age group.

ADOLESCENT GROWTH AND DEVELOPMENT

Various definitions of adolescence have been proposed. Eisen (1984) describes definitions as being aimed at biological research issues, social or interpersonal questions and cultural consider-ations. The rate and timing of transition from childhood through adolescence to adulthood is influenced by different cultures in many differing ways. In most Western societies, however, the adolescent period of development is generally accepted to be those years between 10 and 20 years. A broadly accepted definition of adolescence, as Brook (1985) describes, is the process of growing up, that is the period between childhood and maturity. It encompasses not only the physical changes of puberty but also the emotional, psychological and social differences between adults and children.

In medical terms, adolescents are generally badly catered for as, on the whole, this age group is a healthy section of the population. Should the adolescent run into health problems, such problems usually fall between the expertise of the paediatrician and the various specialities of adult medicine. The World Health Organisation (WHO), through its Division of Maternal and Child Health, set up in 1984 a study group on young people and Health for All by the year 2000. The report of the study, entitled 'Young People's Health – a Challenge for Society', contains a wealth of material and an analysis of the state of adolescent health in the developed and developing world. Great emphasis is placed in this report on the basic needs for advancement in adolescent medicine. This was the first time that an international agency had made such a statement.

THE IMPACT OF CANCER ON THE ADOLESCENT

Adolescents with cancer face not only the tasks of normal growth and development but also the many tasks involved in dealing with their illness. Cancer treatments result in undesirable changes that may cause stress and poor body image at a time when self-esteem and a positive body image are all-important.

The adolescent who is not accepted as he wants to be may use the effects of treatment as a reason for low self-esteem – 'I'm not popular because I have lost my hair due to the treatment'. Alopecia is perhaps one of the most devastating consequences of treatment for the adolescent. For the female, it signifies a loss of feminity and to the male a loss of sex appeal. Wilburn (1980) found that to the adolescent, hair loss was viewed in some cases as being so repulsive that treatment was refused.

Modern surgical techniques and advancement in the use of chemotherapy and radiotherapy have decreased the number of amputations following the diagnosis of bone tumours. However, in some cases amputation may still be warranted. Disfigurement and change in physical appearance can cause the adolescent to withdraw from peers, refuse to continue with educational activities and become isolated. Plumb and Holland (1974) state that, to the adolescent, such side-effects of treatment may be much more alarming than the threat of death itself. The threat of death is fully understood by adolescent patients and is often recognised by their peers as well. This may make friendships difficult as in today's society a mutual discomfort with the issue of death is likely.

The diagnosis of cancer, therefore, imposes stress on the adolescent who is striving to develop independence, identity and a functional role in society. Autonomy will be limited as dependence on parents for care and, in some cases, financial support is imposed. There will also be forced dependency on health workers. Indentity will be impaired, self-esteem will alter as the disease, its treatment and subsequent side-effects cause changes in body image. Sexual identity and sexual function may be influenced. The effects upon the adolescent's functional role in society are numerous and may include a delay in education, fear of unemployment, marriage prospects and limited lifestyle options.

NURSING CARE

All nurses will have gone through adolescence, some with more difficulty than others. In order to care effectively for the adolescent, nurses need to evaluate and settle the issues of their own adolescence and guard against over-identification that they know what the adolescent is feeling. The world in which today's adolescents live is entirely different from the one in which many nurses were adolescents. A nurse treating the adolescent as an equal and whose input is valuable can usually win his confidence. However, because this age group is not always certain of its own values, a nurse's efforts to discuss intimate issues, such as self-image and sexuality, may meet with hostility. Such hostility, if understood and not interpreted as a personal attack, enables the nurse to deal with the problem rationally and calmly.

Nursing Care – at Diagnosis

Koocher and O'Malley (1981) investigated the psychological, medical and life problems of people who were treated successfully for cancer during childhood and adolescence. The question of whether to tell or not to tell was addressed. They and other researchers advocate openness. In recent years, this approach has been adopted by most professionals involved in the treatment and care of the child and adolescent with cancer. This is due in part to a greater understanding that the adolescent cannot be protected from awareness of the serious nature of the illness. As a more honest and open approach is adopted, the question is not whether to tell or not but a question of how the adolescent and his family can be helped to come to terms with the diagnosis and treatment of cancer.

One factor which has been identified as having a significant effect in increasing a positive input at the time of diagnosis is the reaction of others immediately after the adolescent has been informed (Donovan and Pierce, 1976). The response of medical staff, nurses and immediate family seems to be far more important than the severity of the disease itself. Donovan and Pierce state that it makes all the difference in the world if painful facts about oneself are first realised in a friendly and accepting atmosphere.

Honesty is a most important quality when the adolescent and his family are confronted with the diagnosis of cancer. Such honesty should never be without hope, but false optimism may destroy a nurse/patient relationship. As previously mentioned, a nurse needs to recognise the coping mechanisms employed by adolescents. Young people are often angry and show it. Nurses and other health care professionals are a reminder of their illness and anger will be directed towards them. This reaction should be accepted as a healthy reaction. Depression may also be experienced; nurses should avoid a jocular, over-friendly response to depression or anger. A warm sensitivity and a willingness to listen is much more effective.

Family Response to Diagnosis

At diagnosis, nurses need to be aware of the adolescent and his family's response. It is not unusual for family members to attempt to protect each other from painful information. Initially it may be necessary for nurses and health professionals to accept this coping strategy on behalf of family members as they come to terms with the diagnosis and proposed treatment. Gradually, as the diagnosis is accepted and treatment plans understood, it is essential for nursing staff to assist family members and patient to adopt an honest and open sharing of the joys and sorrows that the diagnosis and treatment may bring.

Siblings' understanding of the patient's diagnosis will depend on their age at the time. There is a paucity of research on the siblings of children with cancer. In a retrospective study, Gogan et al (1977) interviewed siblings and report that in general they minimised the impact of the illness and described some feelings of sibling rivalry.

More recently, Spinetta et al (1981) looked at siblings' responses to their brother's or sister's cancer treatment. The results of their study support the fundamental hypothesis that siblings suffer as much and probably more than the patient in unattended emotional responses to the disease and treatment.

The question of how a child or adolescent's long-term illness influences family communication patterns has also been addressed. In an early study, Cobb (1956) reported that parents may not be available to their well children because of the patient's hospitalisation and hospital appointments. Siblings' loneliness and a lack of a structured environment with unknown boundaries can result.

Given support and guidance from knowledgeable nursing staff, all family members can be helped if their individual needs and concerns are not ignored. Continuity with nursing staff seems to help since the patient and family learn to trust and feel comfortable with someone they see on a regular basis. An important nursing role involves the teaching of not only the patient but also parents and other family members about the implication of diagnosis and the rationale of therapy and expected side effects. When considering information to be given to brothers and sisters, nursing staff must work with parents and decide on how best to offer information that is appropriate and age-related. Too often, reports tell of family problems which stem from family members protecting each other and not sharing information with one another honestly.

Nursing Care during Treatment

Adolescents are able to think in abstract terms. Over the years, they have had many learning opportunities and tend to seek out information as they require it. When faced with the diagnosis of cancer and subsequent treatment, adolescents will want to know about diagnostic procedures. The most appropriate way to let an adolescent know that information is available and may be beneficial to them is to say just that.

Generally this age group copes better with investigative procedures if they know why they are being undertaken. Wear et al (1982) state that the preparation of the adolescent may rest not so much on outlining the behaviour required during the procedure as it does on the reasons the procedure needs to be done. In preparation for diagnostic procedures and treatment, the adolescent should be included in conferences with the family, medical and nursing teams to discuss the implications and plans for treatment. An adolescent patient will more than likely want to retain control over what happens to his body although some prefer not to know if the findings of investigations or the treatment plan are too threatening. It is, therefore, essential to ascertain the purpose of questions before giving a direct answer.

It must be remembered that treatment for the cancer may take place over several years. It is, therefore, essential that trust and loyalty is established between the adolescent, his family and health professionals. If trust is not established, unnecessary anxieties and problems may arise. The watchwords for the best adolescent and family care are *stability* and *teamwork*. Ideally, one senior physician should be the adolescent's key doctor throughout the treatment. Similarly, a primary nurse should be the key person to coordinate patient and family care. Given the complexity of diagnostic procedures and current cancer treatments, patient care should be coordinated through a comprehensive cancer centre.

During the treatment phase, it may be necessary for the adolescent to spend time in hospital. This will, of course, depend on the diagnosis and planned treatment. Should hospitalisation be necessary, the question as to where the adolescent is cared for requires addressing. Perhaps the question is more to do with the approach staff have towards the adolescent as discussed previously than the actual physical area.

The needs of adolescents are different from those of both children and adults. Ideally, adolescents should be nursed together. The overemphasis on illness generally found in adult wards is not appropriate to adolescents, whereas in the paediatric ward, their seemingly inexplicable mood swings and ambivalence can make them less appealing than younger children. Yet their need for comfort and understanding is just as great.

The need for privacy, opportunities to discuss and understand the nature of the illness and emotional problems and the ability to maintain contact with family and friends are issues which must concern those caring for adolescents in hospital. Parents, as with younger children, should be able to visit at any time and stay overnight. Siblings and friends should be encouraged and welcomed to visit.

Where possible, the adolescent should be encouraged to participate in planning his hospital day. If chemotherapy is to be given, the timing can be discussed with the patient. He may prefer that the treatment is given after his friends have visited. A flexible approach from staff will indicate to the adolescent that they are willing for him to have some control. This in turn will assist in maintaining a positive self-image on behalf of the patient.

Do we include the adolescent as much as is realistically possible, as much as developmentally we realise the adolescent can hear and understand? Adolescents generally want to be in control of their own care; the more they are actively involved, the more cooperative they become. Accepting this requires nurses and other health care professionals to adopt a flexible approach.

Rigid rules and regulations in the hospital setting will only serve to create unnecessary anxieties for the adolescent. When asked how he attempted to gain control over what happened to him in hospital, an adolescent with cancer answered:

- Now that I've been in and out of hospital a few times, I know which veins are good and which are bad for my chemotherapy. I tell the doctor or the nurse which one to use. They get to try twice and then I ask for someone else.

Not only do these patients decide which vein and which doctor or nurse can be involved, they will also share this information with newly diagnosed adolescents and children.

Adolescents require more individual freedom to move about and to make independent decisions than younger children. However, they need a well-structured environment, one that is more structured than for adult patients. Adolescents will be less likely to test known limits when the consequences are known. For example, a walk in the hospital grounds may only be granted if the adolescent wears outdoor clothes.

Most adolescents are concerned about the adequacy of hospital meals. This concern about meals, common to the healthy adolescent, is exaggerated when the individual is ill and in an environment over which he has no control. Although there is some difference of opinion as to whether food likes and dislikes should be catered for, new food patterns should not be insisted upon. What is important is that he should have adequate nutrition and fluid intake.

Side-effects of chemotherapy and radiotherapy will affect the adolescent's desire for food. A flexible approach to mealtimes and, if possible, allowing him the use of the ward kitchen, will give the adolescent the freedom to prepare his own meals and snacks as desired.

The manner in which the hospitalisation of the adolescent patient is handled by medical and nursing staff determines to a large extent whether the patient's self-image will be kept intact, and whether the medical management of his disease will be successful. As a general rule it is best to be honest with adolescents, incorporating supportive remarks into discussions: 'Has the diagnosis of cancer made you feel angry? People your age tell me it does.' A question phrased in this manner indicates that it is normal to feel angry and he is not on his own.

Brook (1985) states that most adolescents complain that they are misunderstood and, from their point of view, this may well be true since many of the problems of adolescents are actually the problems of the adults who are having the deal with them.

EDUCATION

As the prospects of cure for adolescents with cancer increase, the long-term consequences of treatment and the quality of life experienced by survivors must assume greater importance. Early return to formal education for those of school age is of considerable importance both educationally and socially. To facilitate the adolescent's return, teachers require information about the types of cancer adolescents may develop and the specific implications for schooling. Holmes and Holmes (1975) found that the effects of school absenteeism are reported by long-term survivors to be among the most important consequences of having had cancer. High rates of absenteeism found among children and adolescents with cancer are partly explained by visits to clinics and periods of hospitalisation. Charlton et al (1986) have shown that children and adolescents encounter many difficulties when returning to school following diagnosis. Anxieties and embarrassment arising from their illness, together with the development of a dependent protective relationship between the adolescent and parent, may reinforce absence from school.

The adolescent's return to the classroom may present challenges for his school friends. It is important to be honest with peers regarding their friend's illness in order to allay fears and rumours. The adolescent will be acutely aware of any change in attitude on the part of the teacher or his school friends. This in turn may lead him to adopt the 'sick role' as a means of opting out in order to cope.

Stevens et al (1988) surveyed the extent to which professional contact is fostered between children's cancer centres and the education service. Results show that efforts to achieve contact between cancer centres and educational services in the United Kingdom are variable. Centres acknowledged the importance of information for schools and written information was available. However, only a few addressed issues such as explaining that the child or adolescent is usually aware of their own diagnosis, and that acute medical problems rarely occur when the patient has returned to school. Patients should be encouraged to return to school as soon as possible and to participate in their normal activities to the extent that their physical condition permits. This return to school requires active discussions with anxious school teachers and with potentially protective parents. Nurses are in a prime position to discuss rehabilitative activities for the adolescent such as a return to school with parents and school teachers. School teachers frequently make contact with the hospitalised adolescent and his parents. Nursing staff should use such contacts to answer appropriate questions and offer pertinent information. Charlton (1989) carried out a study funded by the Cancer Research Campaign to find out what school teachers knew about cancer. The study highlighted that teachers wanted specific information from a 'medical source' about how to care for a child with cancer returning to school.

Overall, the author summarised that teachers needed information about cancer in general, a chance to examine their own feelings and to understand the reality of the current status of treatment and curability for all cancers, but especially for childhood ones.

EMPLOYMENT

Most of the literature on the subject of employment and employment discrimination against recovered patients with cancer has focused on adults rather than adolescents or former child patients with cancer. Employers who have responded to studies about their attitudes to employing survivors of cancer reflect deep fears of cancer. Courts et al (1976) found that 61 per cent of employers cited the fear of increases in insurance premiums as a justification for not hiring cancer survivors. Other reasons mentioned for not employing survivors of cancer were fears about decreased productivity, excessive sick leave and the possibility of the employee's sudden death.

Koocher and O'Malley (1981) state that the United States' military policy on applicants with a history of cancer could not be clearer – automatic disqualification. The reason given for this policy is the need to have as fit a military force as possible.

Employment and insurance coverage seem to present significant problems for many adolescent survivors of cancer. There is a need therefore to educate potential employers and dispel unfounded myths about cancer. And insurance underwriters require more information in order more accurately to conform to current survival expectations.

Marriage Prospects

Sexuality and the ability to produce a child are two areas that trouble adolescents. Fears about reproductive capabilities need to be shared with the health care team. Future spouses or sex partners may also be uncertain about the ability of the cured individual to participate in sexual relations. Frequently, the concern is a psychological one, although in some cases a physical or physiological factor may be present.

Some chemotherapeutic agents are gonadotoxic, causing amenorrhoea and decreased spermatogenesis. Even so, some former patients have successfully parented a child. Radiotherapy to the gonads does cause sterility and patients must be informed of this. Sperm banking for the male adolescent requires consideration. It must be stressed, however, that cancer therapies do not impair sexual function.

As the adolescent survives and enters the adult world, rehabilitative consultation is required. They should know of the problems they may face and advice given as to how problems may be overcome. Clearly as nurses arm themselves with knowledge of survivors' potential problems, they can participate in rehabilitative services by assisting the patient and his family to seek appropriate assistance, guidance and help.

SUMMARY

Adolescence is a time of tremendous change, characterised by conflicting high and low periods as the individual seeks to find his own identity. The adolescent is rebellious, inconsistent, uncertain, grown-up one minute, childish the next. How he appears in the eyes of others is all-important. Opinions and attitudes of his peers are important for his sense of self-confidence and worth.

Minor blemishes can assume great importance and doubts about a positive body image. The impact of a diagnosis of cancer on this age group can be devastating (Figure 9.1).

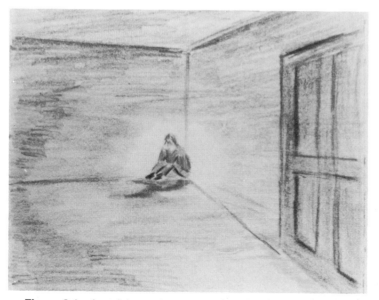

Figure 9.1   An adolescent expresses how he feels in a drawing

Adolescents demand from nurses and other health care professionals honest and accurate information about their illness. Nurses must promote efforts to reduce the prevalent over-emphasis on physical appearance in our culture. Careful preparation of individuals for events in which self-concept and self-image may change is important.

Adolescent patients must be cared for not as children or adults but as an age group with specific needs. It is important to understand their development and how medical problems affect their mood, behaviour and coping. It is a special time in their lives, both psychologically and biologically. They need and deserve a special kind of understanding.

References

Brook C G D (1985) *All about Adolescence.* Chichester: John Wiley and Sons.

Charlton A (1989) What does a school teacher know? In *Cancer Nursing: a Revolution in Care*, Pritchard A P (ed.), pp. 29-32. London: Macmillan.

Charlton A, Pearson D and Morris Jones P H (1986) Children's return to school after treatment for solid tumours. *Society of Scientific Medicine:* **22:** 1337-1346.

Cobb B (1956) Psychological impact of long-term illness and death of a child on the family circle, *Journal of Paediatrics.* **45**(6): 746.

Cohen M and Wellisch D (1978) Living in limbo. Psychological intervention in families with a cancer patient. *American Journal of Psychotherapy,* **32:** 561-571.

Courts S, Rodov M and Wilcom M (1976) Attitudes of employers and cancer patients towards patients' work ability. Rehabilitative programme, National Cancer Institute Contract. Pittsburgh: Centre for Health Systems Studies.

Donovan M and Pierce S (1976) Identity and body image, *Cancer Care Nursing.* New York: Appleton-Century-Crofts.

Eisen P (1984) Adolescence: coping strategies and vulnerabilities. *International Journal of Adolescent Medicine & Health,* **2:** 107-115.

Gogan J R, Koocher G P, Foster D J and O'Malley J E (1977) Impact of childhood cancer on siblings. *Health and Social Work,* **2**(1): 41-57.

Holmes H A and Holmes F F (1975) After ten years what are the handicaps and lifestyles of children treated for cancer? *Clinical Paediatrics,* **14:** 819-823.

Klopovich P M and Clancy B J (1985) Sexuality and the adolescent with cancer. *Seminars in Oncology Nursing,* **1**(1): 42-48.

Koocher G P and O'Malley J E (1981) *The Damocles Syndrome. Psychological Consequences of Surviving Childhood Cancer.* New York: McGraw-Hill.

Plumb M and Holland J (1974) Cited in Koocher and O'Malley, *The Damocles Syndrome*, p. 8. New York: McGraw-Hill.

Spinetta J J, McLare H H, Deasey-Spinetta P M, Kung F H, Schwartz D B and Hartman G A (1981) *Responses of siblings to their brother's or sister's cancer treatment. A three-year study.* Unpublished manuscript. San Diego State University.

Stevens M C G, Kaye J I, Kenwood C F and Man J R (1988) Facts for teachers of children with cancer. *Archives of Disease in Childhood*, **63**: 456-458.

Wear E T, Covey J and Brush M (1982) Facilitating children's adaptation to intrusive procedures. In: *Nursing Care of the Child with Cancer*, Fochtman D and Foley G V (eds.), p. 70. Boston: Little, Brown.

Wilburn J (1980) Sexual development and body image in the adolescent with cancer. In: *Adolescent Medicine: Present and Future Concepts*, Rigg C and Shaun W (eds.), p. 171. Chicago: Yearbook Medical Publishers.

10
The Child with Cancer in the Community

THE CHILD IN THE COMMUNITY

In the 1980s, more children had survived cancer than at any time in the past. Take, for example, the survival rate of children treated for leukaemia following a recent clinical trial, which finished in November 1986. This trial showed that out of 829 patients introduced to this treatment protocol, 537 child patients were surviving after five years. It is these children, surviving in the community, who need the early intervention of community support at the time of diagnosis. Research has shown that community services are lacking for the general paediatric population. Hence a child with cancer with his or her special needs is less likely to receive adequate community support.

Looking broadly at the community, one has to ponder a little and consider whom it comprises. Apart from the immediate and extended family unit, the child and family are in contact with many other people within a very short time. From the community angle, first one has to look at the involvement of the primary health care team.

Role of the General Practitioner (GP)

It is a well-known fact that a GP will encounter perhaps only one child with cancer throughout his practising career. The child and parent may have visited the GP's surgery several times before the child is referred to the District General Hospital or a specialist centre. This provokes a certain amount of anger and resentment on the part of the parent towards the GP. To help the family regain their confidence in the GP, it is important to explain the rarity of childhood cancer to the family, and to re-establish early contact with the GP. Although on confirmation of the diagnosis medical staff at the specialist centre will inform the GP this may take several weeks.

The task of early liaison with the GP can be undertaken by the specialist hospital community paediatric or the community based paediatric nurse. She can provide the necessary information regarding the child's diagnosis, treatment plan and problems relating to possible side-effects of treatment. This would alert the GP into making appropriate arrangements for the family to have easy access to his services which in turn would lessen the parents' anxiety and help to gain their confidence. Regular liaison also encourages the GP to keep in touch with the specialist centre and to make occasional visits to the unit.

Role of the Health Visitor

Health visitors can play an important role in giving the child and family continuous psychosocial support throughout the child's illness. Generally, the health visitor is viewed as looking after 'healthy children' of 0–5 years of age. She may give adequate support to mentally and physically handicapped children, but when she encounters a child with cancer she may find herself avoiding the family because of her own lack of knowledge about the diagnosis and treatment.

If the child is under five years at the time of diagnosis, the health visitor is more likely to know the family than if the child is older. The hospital community liaison nurse can establish early contact with the health visitor, so that a home visit is made soon after the child's discharge from hospital.

In the case of an older child, the health visitor may need to make contact with the family, and gain their confidence so that the family will identify her contact as beneficial. There will also be the need to contact the child's school and the school nurse.

As the health visitor is expert at monitoring the under-five year olds' normal developmental milestones, her observation and early detection of a child's slowness in any development area would enable her to refer the child to the appropriate agencies, e.g. portage system assessment for under five's with a brain tumour, where development may be hindered because of the anatomical position of the tumour.

The health visitor can assess the family's needs and organise practical help such as voluntary baby-sitters, home help or social services worker where necessary. For the parents she can help by just listening and giving them time to express their views and concerns.

Role of the District Nurse

District nurses over the years have been looked upon as caring for the elderly in the community. However, recently district nurses are becoming involved in caring for the young, and in a few areas of the country, paediatric district nursing services are being set up. The district nurse's involvement in the care of the child with cancer may be for the child who has undergone surgery and either the District General Hospital or the GP will have requested services from the district nurse for home care.

When required, the district nurse is called upon to supervise the parents with the care of central venous lines, but as most district nurses are unable due to local policies to give intravenous therapy, this causes a great deal of frustration both to the nurse and to the parents. Hopefully, in time the need for such training will be realised and given appropriately, as children are discharged much sooner from hospital, frequently with a central venous lines in situ.

Role of School Nurse and Community Paediatrician

In recent years the school nurse has played an important part, as she is involved in the care of the child with cancer at school. Her function is that of 'health educator' and of assessing the child's needs at school. She will alert the community paediatrician who will contact the GP or the specialist centre to obtain adequate information to help the child settle in school or, if necessary, to arrange home tuition. If the child/family needs psychological help, this can be initiated by the community paediatrician.

Other Agencies

The community social worker may have to be involved in instances where family stresses, financial or otherwise, are increased, or when the care of other children in the family is at risk due to the parents' need to spend time with their sick child.

Macmillan, Marie Curie, Rupert and CLIC Nurses, funded by charitable organisations, play a major role in supporting the child and the family through the terminal phase of the child's illness. If the family is living some distance from the child's treatment centre, the hospital liaison nurse or the community paediatric nurse needs to establish early contact with the various supporting agencies before the parents take their child home. Early discharge planning in such instances is essential.

EDUCATION

Education plays an important part in the formative years of all children's lives. If they have started on a good footing, liking their school, teachers and peers this environment is conducive to good educational achievements, whether it be academic or practical. In this cycle of events, if the child is faced with a life-threatening illness, this will affect his/her educational achievements to the extent that the child may seek to opt out of the system. 'Opting out' may be as a result of feeling 'different' owing to the illness, side-effects from the treatment and changes in self-image. For a young child starting playgroup, nursery or infants school, it can be stressful, first because of separation from the parents and, secondly, for the parents as they allow their child who has cancer into an unknown area.

To assist the child to overcome this anxiety and help him adjust into the school environment, it is important to liaise with playgroups, nursery schools and schools. With the parents' permission the community liaison nurse is able to make contact with the school. The aims of such visits are:

- To give correct information regarding the child's illness and treatment plan.
- To offer information about the child's physical changes and how to cope with specific situations, e.g. following hair loss the hair will re-grow.
- To give information regarding possible infection especially problems related to chicken-pox and measles and to give clear guidelines on what action to take.
- The need for flexibility on the part of the school while the child is undergoing treatment. Lack of energy is to be expected during this period, and teachers need to understand that this will improve once the child has finished treatment.

Teacher's Role

The teacher is able to deal with the child's illness from the information gained from the specialist nurse as follows:

- The teacher will be equipped to explain the child's absence from the class and to remember the child during school activities.
- Prepare other children about the physical changes of the ill child such as:

> - Loss of hair during treatment and the reasons why
> - Changes in weight – loss or gain
> - Loss of a limb through surgery or a defective limb where the tumour is being treated.

- To be aware of the child being teased in school – normally the child's peer group is protective towards the child, but other children may not be so.
- While the child is hospitalised, it is important for the teacher to keep in touch with the child and the family. In addition, it helps if school friends are encouraged to keep in touch by writing or visiting.
- After treatment, it is important to welcome back the child as 'normal'.
- The teacher must alert other parents in the child's class to his or her vulnerability to infectious diseases, and give them explicit guidelines on what action to take in such circumstances.

Normally children up to the age of seven years settle back into school routine fairly quickly, on either a long- or short-term basis. Seven- to thirteen-year-olds are acutely aware of their self-image. Changes are frequently noticed and they are often teased by other children. The adolescent may have witnessed a few deaths during his stay in hospital and is aware of the potential fatality of his own disease. The choice of opting out of the education system can easily set in with this age group, especially with those who have played truant prior to their illness. It is a major hurdle to go back to school, but once achieved they are usually accepted and able to regain their confidence. Peer group support can be variable during this period.

However, some adolescents feel that nobody understands how they feel, having cancer and undergoing aggressive treatment. There is a distinct lack of empathy from their peers and only a few remain supportive and understanding. Long-standing friendships are often lost if there has been a long absence from school. This can lead to long-term psychological and emotional damage.

Home Tuition

Children who are subjected to aggressive chemotherapy regimes at few-weekly intervals over a six-month period or longer, or those who have to undergo bone marrow transplantation

(BMT), miss long periods of schooling. The hospital teacher will need to liaise with the local education authority to arrange home tuition once the treatment plan is known. This will enable the child to keep up with his school work and may prevent him from falling behind the other children on his return to school.

In exceptional cases, where the child is very conscious of the change in his body image (e.g. loss of hair), home tuition may need to be arranged giving the child time to come to terms with the changes he faces on the understanding that a return to school must take place once the child feels happier about himself.

HOME VISITS

Therapy for childhood cancer has become more aggressive and complex, and at the same time increasingly more successful. The approach to care for the child with cancer can roughly be divided into three stages:

- The time of diagnosis and administration of therapy.
- The time of remission and anticipated good health.
- If the treatments are unsuccessful, the period leading to the death of the child.

Each of these requires different kinds of support, which cannot always be provided by members of the community, and are usually provided by the multidisciplinary team from the oncology centre.

Lengthy discussions about the child's disease and treatment assist with accurate and appropriate care planning. Following diagnosis and initial treatment the child may be discharged home after three to six weeks. An essential part of care for the child and family is to receive a home visit from a specialist nurse.

A home visit provides an opportunity for families to continue to seek new information and to clarify recently acquired information about their child's disease and treatment.

The dramatic increase in the number of children surviving cancer has created the need for nurses who visit the child's home who specialise in helping the family adjust to life, the diagnosis of cancer, its treatment and in the long term, follow-up care for the surviving patient in the community.

Objectives and Nurse's Assessment of Home Visit

Before embarking on a home visit, the nurse must realise that each family has individual needs, and some of the factors to be considered are social, cultural, religious and language. Generally, the kinds of services that the home nurse provides are assessment of the family and their coping mechanisms, assessment of the home environment, teaching of procedures, patient advocacy, health education and supportive counselling.

Discussion of the Diagnosis

This is vital, as in many instances families have been disorientated by the hospital environment and the shock of their child's diagnosis. Clarification of medical terminology may be necessary where perhaps the word 'tumour' is not equated to cancer due to language difficulties.

Parents'/Child's Understanding of the Disease Process and Treatment Protocols

When parents ask, they need to know that although two children may have a similar diagnosis, tumour bulk, site and plus/minus distant metastases at presentation determine an important part of the eventual outcome of the child's illness.

Assessment of Parents' Information Gained during the Period of Hospitalisation

Parents need clear instructions on how to look after a Hickman or Broviac line, and, likewise, a guideline to follow if the child shows signs of infection due to a low blood count, or is in direct contact with measles or chicken-pox.

Family Dynamics – Assessment of Effects on Parents, Siblings and Extended Family Members

Taking their child home after initial hospitalisation is a frightening prospect for any parent. The family has to make adjustments to their lifestyles, as their life revolves around the 'sick' child. Home visits by the hospital community nurse or a paediatric community nurse provide a good opportunity to help parents so that they begin to look upon their child as 'normal'. They will gain confidence in allowing their child to be regarded as 'normal' as the child responds to treatment and shows improvement in his physical and emotional state. Eventually, the aim is for parents to become less dependent on the unit and become competent advocates for their child's health needs.

Siblings

Siblings are encouraged to visit freely in a 'family-centred care' unit, yet experience and studies reveal that certain stresses are unique to healthy brothers and sisters of a child with cancer. The feeling of abandonment through recurring periods of separation, jealousy, resentment and rivalry in younger children to feelings of guilt and deep distress, learning difficulties/lack of concentration in older siblings are some of the phenomena. The child with cancer becomes an object of natural total concern and parents should be made aware of the 'needs' of healthy children. Home visits provide an opportunity to reassure parents, healthy brothers and sisters when necessary, and to make suggestions or appropriate referrals that will assist the family to cope. For example, there may be a need to involve the services of a child psychologist.

Any childhood illness will cause stress within a relationship, but a child with a life-threatening condition tests interpersonal relationship to the limit. Parents are often surprised at their reactions as individuals to their child's illness, and invariably find it difficult to talk about such feelings. The home environment provides a unique opportunity for letting parents express views and the visiting nurse provides a 'listening ear' in a counselling role. If the partnership has been under stress before the child's illness, and parents are suddenly placed in a position of caring for their child as equals, the nurse can help them to recognise certain strengths in such a relationship. Single parents face double the stress in looking after the child with cancer. Their special needs have to be recognised and appropriate psychological support input is essential.

During the home visit it is important to ascertain who are the members of the extended family, friends and spiritual support the family has. In today's nuclear family concept, the grandparents are often living away from the family and the parents do not want to 'burden' them with their problems. In many instances, good friends and the church support the family through their difficult periods. The parents need reassurance not to feel guilty in accepting a 'helping hand'. Practical help such as a neighbour cooking a meal for the family is of great value.

NURSING THE TERMINALLY ILL CHILD AT HOME

Death and dying provoke all kinds of emotions in a person, and these are intensified when one is faced with a dying child. As care-givers, we have to work through our own feelings and emotions about the dying process and eventual death. This will assist nurses to support the families when they are going through one of the potentially most stressful and poignant experiences that a family can encounter. When it becomes evident that a child's disease is not responding, and active/curative treatment has to cease, the child's care during the terminal phase has to be discussed with the parents. Such discussion will initially be with the physician and the home care nurse, and the family is given a choice of home or hospital care. Through experience it is becoming evident that most parents opt to care for their dying child at home. In order to achieve maximum comfort for the child and the family, the nurse needs to assess home care resources.

Home Care Resources

At the terminal phase of the child's illness, parents are confronted with a period of unknown duration and their role as parents is threatened. One parent wrote that 'anticipatory grief' tests the individual, the marriage, the siblings, the grandparents and other relatives, and one's own faith.

There are important issues that need to be considered and discussed with the parents. First, is it possible to provide home care for the child? Here the care-givers and parental capabilities have to be carefully considered. Through experience it is a well-established fact that parents care for their child admirably with minimum support. Secondly, desirability has to be considered. Here the lack of support from extended family or friends puts an extra stress on the parents. In addition, there is the worry of the effect of the dying child on healthy siblings. Therefore, the choice of the child/family returning to the hospital must be emphasised. Such a dialogue builds a trusting relationship between the nurse and the parents, which in turn leads to open communication. The two fears that are regularly uppermost in parents' minds are:

- Uncontrollable symptoms, especially pain.
- What would happen at the time of actual death (i.e. fear of the unknown)?

The family needs the assurance from the home care nurse that twenty-four hours' back-up service is going to be available and will be provided as and when necessary. With the knowledge that such a service is available, parents never abuse the system.

Psychologically, the parents have been dependent on the unit staff throughout the child's active treatment period; their reluctance to accept unfamiliar outside nursing help is understandable. From the practical point of view, if the family lives some distance from the treatment centre, early intervention from Paediatric Community Nursing Services, including Macmillan or Marie Curie Nurses and the GP, is important. Early liaison with the primary health care team and relevant agencies will facilitate the availability of the team within twenty-four hours of the child's discharge from the hospital. If within travelling distance, it is important for the home care nurse to meet the team. By doing so it is hoped that the child and his parents will have confidence in the services provided by the community.

Nurses in a paediatric setting have to remember certain home care criteria:

- In the home environment the parent is the primary care-giver.
- The nurse is a facilitator in achieving the child's peaceful death.
- The physician needs to be approachable, available and flexible. The flexibility of prescribing adequate and necessary medication and for the GP to use home care nurse or specialist unit as a resource.

Role of the Home Care Nurse

The physical, psychological and emotional support required by families and children who are dying at home clearly falls into the capability of professional nursing. It is vital for the home care nurse to follow certain guidelines which will assist her in maximising the child's and the family's comfort.

- Pain control is a paramount issue in everybody's mind, not least the parents who are caring for their child twenty-four hours a day. Oral analgesia is very effective in most children until the time when the child is unable to swallow. Subcutaneous or intravenous pain control will then become necessary, the drug given via a syringe pump. Parents may have to be taught about dosages and the frequency and administration of drugs via the pump. They soon become proficient at such a task, which gives them a degree of control over the situation.

Other potential symptoms such as nausea, vomiting, constipation and mouth ulcers should be assessed regularly and if necessary treated accordingly. When the child needs blood products for symptom control, arrangements for this therapy to be given at home helps to avoid or minimise hospital visits. Such a service offers both physical and psychological comfort to the child and his family.

- For a child to die with dignity, physical comforts must be assessed and provided for. Wheelchair, commode, sheepskin or a special mattress should be readily available to lessen unnecessary worry for the child and parent. If the child's pain control necessitates the use of pump for a length of time, his mobility must be maintained.
- Nursing the child on a settee or in his own bed downstairs in the centre of family activities helps to create a secure environment for the child. For such a purpose, the parents usually have to make certain physical changes to their living accommodation. Such an environment encourages the siblings to participate in the child's care and play activities.
- The nurse has to assess, act and evaluate her actions as the child's condition deteriorates over a period of time. It is important that continuity of care is maintained and the nurse is accessible twenty-four hours a day.
- When the child is nursed at home it becomes a daily activity for the brothers and sisters to participate in his care. Yet as parents are totally engrossed in looking after the dying child, their healthy children's emotional demands may go unheeded. The nurse is in the prime position to assist parents to realise the needs of their healthy children. Help and support of the extended family members, mainly grandparents, can be a great source of comfort for parents and healthy children alike. However, they also require support in coming to terms with their anticipated grief.
- Parents may want to nurse their child at home for as long as possible, but do not want their child to die at home. The nurse must remain in close contact with the physician, and through her vigilance and the doctor's assessment, the child can be moved into the hospital at the right time.

- Parents need clear guidelines as to whom to call when the child dies, especially at night, if the nurse or doctor is not present.

Parents worry that their child may confront them directly about death and dying. Children have various means of communicating their feelings on death without direct questioning. Here is an example of a fourteen-year-old girl who dictated this poem to her mother just a few weeks before she died at home.

The Wilderness

At the end of the day
The clouds break away,
They form tumbling boulders of soft grey smoke and dust
Evaporating into the beautiful pink sunset's cooling rays.
The lion cubs, lionesses and lion bowl around playfully
———— Under the shaded whispering fir trees
And the silent cackles and laughs of the hyaenas
Beat around the bush.

About the only sound you'll never hear
Around your glowing log campfire
Is the off-distant sound
Of traffic, a Jeep or gunshots
To spoil the last dying figments
Of the dissolving day.

4 June 1987

The clouds tumbled into the hot diminishing skies
Evaporating into the hot dying sun
A drizzle
And then the rain poured down,
This time needing no shelter at all.
The gulleys, crevices and cracks filled up
And were replenished
With a new life.

The cubs cheerfully plodded around
And splashed about in the new, cool water holes
Splashing and playing,
And the birds began to chatter
Bringing a whole new life
Into the undying, undrying wilderness beyond.

11 June 1987
Gemma Marshall

After the death of a child, the family disassociates from members of the hospital staff and tries to readjust to previously established family patterns. The memories of having done the very best that they could for their child will help to sustain the family during the time of transition. Parents as individuals have to grieve separately and one has to give them time, space and support as necessary.

In conclusion, as the number of long-term survivors increases, the importance of adequate psychosocial support for children and families in the community needs to be recognised and made available.

Further Reading

Ferguson J and Hobbie W (1985) Home visits for the child with cancer. *Nursing Clinics of North America*, **20**(1): 109-115.

Gillespie A (1985) Spotlite on Fife (Macmillan continuing care services). *Senior Nurse*, **3**(6): inside back cover.

Hinds C (1985) The needs of families who care for patients with cancer at home: are we meeting them? *Journal of Advanced Nursing*, **10**(6): 575–581.

Houlton E (1986) The Jacks of all trades. *Senior Nurse*, **5**(2): 24-25.

Kohler J A and Radford M (1985) Terminal care of children dying of cancer – quantity and quality of life. *British Medical Journal*, **291**: 115-116.

Lauer M E and Camitta B M (1980) *Journal of Paediatrics*, **97**(6): 1032-1035.

Lauer M E, Mulhern R K, Hoffman R G and Camitta B M (1986) Utilisation of hospice/home care in paediatric oncology (in USA). *Cancer Nursing*, **9**(3): 102-107.

Martinson I M, Moldow D G, Armstrong G D, Henry W F, Nesbit M E and Kersey J H (1986) Home care for children dying of cancer. *Research in Nursing and Health*, **9**(1): 11-16.

Norman R and Bennett M (1986) Care of the dying child at home: a unique co-operative relationship. *Australian Journal of Advanced Nursing*, **3**(4): 3-16.

Price B J (1979) Caring for the child with cancer: the nurse practitioner. *Cancer Nurse*, **75**(11): 48-50.

Ross A K (1985) Supportive care for families of dying children. *Nursing Clinics of North America*, **20**(2): 457-465.

11
Care of the Terminally Ill Child

PREPARATION

Terminal care can be described as care that prepares someone for death. Preparation should start at the diagnosis of a life-threatening disease or when therapy towards cure is no longer accepted as appropriate. Therapy, therefore, changes direction but should remain equally positive and aim for a good quality of life, however short. The essence of care is to continue with as near-normal routines and lifestyle as possible.

The child's parents, or parent with a relative or friend, should be interviewed by the consultant together with another member of the caring team. This may be the primary nurse, ward sister or someone who has been closely involved in the care of the child. It is difficult to explain to parents, who may have brought a 'well' child to a routine clinic visit, that his illness has returned, the progress of the disease cannot be halted and, this time, there is no curative therapy that can be offered. Since diagnosis the parents may have pushed to the back of their minds the fact that death might be the outcome. Accepting that their aspirations for their child's future will not now be realised is not easy.

THE DECISION

The decision to stop active therapy towards remission or cure can be devastating to parents. Throughout the course of the illness the hospital and staff have become their world, and now they may feel they are being 'rejected' and feel isolated. What about the remote chance of further treatment, couldn't the medical staff try? Opportunities to ask the same questions should be made available. Parents have the rest of their lives to live and need to know that everything possible was done. Hope must not be destroyed entirely, as it is hope that keeps parents going from one day to the next – if not hope of life, then hope of comfort.

How Long?

The last weeks and days are precious to the family and can contribute to the recollection of happy times after the death of their child. One cannot be sure when a child with progressive disease will die – many children have lived to see another Christmas, birthday or week that was thought to be impossible. Although a professional guess may be given about the likelihood of events, there is no certainty.

WHERE TO DIE?

Where the child is finally cared for should be the parents', and if appropriate, the child's decision. It is the role of all involved professionals to provide maximum physical, psychosocial support and guidance. It may be that the child has a 'lot of living to do', if the state of his health allows. There is no reason why a special holiday or activity should not be undertaken. The aim at all times is for the best quality of life, however short.

If the Child Is to Die at Home

The hospital doctor or hospital community liaison nurse, or whoever is responsible in the District Health Authority, or community paediatric nurse should communicate with the general practitioner (GP) as early as possible. This may be the GP's first experience of caring for a dying child at home, and may be stressful personally as well as professionally to the GP. The same is true of the community nurse. Hospital team members should make it clear to community staff that they are available, and if possible the paediatric liaison nurse should meet the community nurse in the child's home to discuss the situation, expectations and plans.

There is an increasing number of hospices throughout the United Kingdom, some of which have facilities for terminally ill children. It may be that the family choose this facility for respite or terminal care rather than the hospital. However, in many cases the length of time the child has between being able to carry on a fairly normal life and his death is relatively short.

If the Child Is to Die in Hospital

As much living as possible should take place in the familiar environment of the home. It is not until the quality of life has deteriorated so that the child has become bed-bound that hospitalisation may become necessary. The hospital environment may be familiar to the parents, but some time may have passed since his last admission and the members of staff may have changed. Hospital is often viewed as a 'safe' place – people accept the child's disabilities there, and his parents will not be totally responsible for his care which can be a relief to them. The role of the nurse is to see that all the needs of the child are met, the core of which is to ensure that parents are able to do as much of that care as they wish or are able. Parents know their child, his habits and routines and are in the best position to meet his needs. They need to believe, after the child's death, that 'we did everything we could'. Accommodation for parents to be resident will allow some control of the situation they face. Their control on the life of their child, which until then has been theirs, particularly with reference to parenting, may be lost during hospitalisation. Participation should therefore give parents a sense of control and involvement in decision-making.

A nurse must be alert to the needs of the parents. This may require encouraging them to eat properly, to get a good night's sleep and to help them in practical as well as supportive ways. Parents need support together and individually, and require to have time together to share feelings and fears, and perhaps even to discuss the funeral. However, some parents may find communication difficult as one may want to talk and the other not. They may not see themselves as important as they concentrate on caring for their child. Without the normal domestic activities of home life time may seem endless, and 'time off duty' if only brief is as important for them as it is for staff. Assuring parents that someone will stay with their child will help them to accept a break more easily. Terminal illness should not prevent a child from having outings in a car or pram, so that for a short time the family can be together in a more normal environment than on a ward. There should be no rules but a flexible approach. An advantage of the hospital environment is the number of people around and available to offer support. A disadvantage is that everyone may believe that someone else is providing the support when each professional is rushing from one urgent task to another. Primary nursing enables one nurse to coordinate care for the child and his family.

Within the hospital many services are available. For example, education and schooling are so much a part of a child's life that dying is no reason to stop providing it, indeed its role in maintaining a 'normal' routine of daily activity is extremely important. If a child is anxious to continue to study for GCSE examinations, although there is no realistic hope of his sitting exams, the teacher must accept the child's wish with commitment and enthusiasm.

The child's approach to dying will be as unique as his or her approach to living (Hall et al, 1982). There are, however, similarities in the understanding of death among children, depending on developmental status (Table 11.1).

Table 11.1 Age-related fears of children and adolescents in relation to death

Age	Fears
1–3 years (toddler)	Separation Immobility No comprehension of death
4–5 years (pre-school)	Separation Darkness Immobility Bodily intrusion Death is reversible
6–11 years (school age)	Loss of control Punishment for wrong-doing Pain Death as a reality
11 years + (adolescent)	Death Unrealised dreams Loss of independence Increased dependence on parents/carers

The role of the dietitian may become increasingly challenging as boredom with food sets in, appetite disappears, vomiting occurs or other such problems arise. 'Filling in time' might be difficult, as the child's attention-span decreases or his activity ability drops as weakness increases. The occupational therapist can help the parent and nurse to provide appliances to make caring easier. The physiotherapist will be involved as the provision of passive exercise and support to weakening muscles will help psychologically as well as physically. Dying does not necessarily mean fewer supportive services but may in fact require more.

Family and friends, especially school friends, should visit freely with the agreement of everyone. As many personal belongings as can reasonably be accommodated from home should be accepted, always considering that the ward area must remain safe for all who occupy it. Family, love and praise, and favourite possessions in a friendly environment provide support and encouragement to the child and his parents.

A birthday close to the end of life can be a happy celebration filled with laughter, visitors and photographs. The effect on everyone, family and carers alike, can temporarily obliterate the sadness of what the future holds.

The care of siblings is as essential as that of the child; it is easy for them to be unthinkingly left out as attention is concentrated on the last days of the child who has already taken so much of the parents' time and love. Even the very young will remember this event all their lives; therefore care of siblings is very important. Has anyone stopped to understand a sibling's altered behaviour, sometimes interpreted as 'naughtiness', which is an expression of his feelings? Feelings of being left out is a very bitter emotion, as is jealousy, because someone else is getting all the attention. He may feel unwanted, unloved and worse may still believe it is all his fault. Simply being present could help him to feel included in the care of his dying brother or sister. Has he had some undivided attention from his parents to ask questions and get answers? If he asks 'Is he going to die?', it would be wrong to deny the event as a strong possibility even to the very young. Children too need the chance to say goodbye. Are grandparents being left out of knowing what is going on? Does anyone know how they feel? A disadvantage in the hospital environment is that the opportunity for family communication may not be as free as at home.

BODY IMAGE

The process of dying can be difficult. Often the child and his family have to become accustomed to ongoing changes in body image such as hair loss, loss of a limb, loss of mobility, body weight loss or gain. Given time, most children adapt to such changes, especially younger ones, but frequently there is not time, as weakness and exhaustion are experienced. Adolescents in particular are very aware of their altered body image and many want to hide away from family and friends. Parents can be even more distressed at changes in the child, and experience difficulties in helping the child to adjust. For them the final memory of their child perhaps on a ventilator can be a very difficult one to forget.

SYMPTOM CONTROL

While many problems require medical attention, the nurse may be the first to detect distressing symptoms.

Pain

If a child says he has a pain, then he has a pain, and he needs relief, but pain can be difficult to measure. Pain has two aspects:

1. The direct aspect of the pain itself – considering how much and in what way normal activities are restricted by the pain are very important in assessment. The type of cry, or how much the child can describe it. Measuring pain is difficult and depending on the child's understanding, the line method may help – *a little* ———————— *a lot*. The child points to a place on the line indicating the degree of pain. Facial expression will also help with the assessment.
2. The indirect aspect of general comfort, restlessness, company, hunger, thirst, constipation, etc.

The degree to which the child can be diverted by something which takes his interest will help guide the need for analgesia, its type, quality and effectiveness. One child may not have pain; another may not complain of it. Should an otherwise unexplained restlessness be removed by analgesia, it is accepted the child had pain. The parents' role in assessing pain is very important and their very presence is of considerable help in alleviating it. If the child understands the severity of the disease, such as 'You have a lump and it is in a position to hurt, and this is what we will do', the severity of the pain may be eased. The method of analgesia varies considerably from one child needing regular paracetamol (60 mg/kg/24 hr × 4), to another needing regular slow-releasing morphine tablets (MST 10 mg b.d. from 2 years of age, doubled at 6 years). Such analgesics as DF118 (dihydro-codeine) have adverse effects on young children and therefore are only considered from 6 years (1 mg/kg/24 hrs, 6-hourly × 4).

Transcutaneous electronic nerve stimulation (TENS) is a 'magic black box' and a non-invasive method of providing relief, when the site of the pain is identified. The stimulator pad is placed over the painful site, the box emits pulses along the nerve conductor. This stimulates the production of endorphines in the spinal cord inhibiting the message of 'pain' to the brain.

Following successful pain control using oral diamorphine, which also has the benefit of producing a sense of well-being, a successful method of administration as the dose requires increase is the use of a subcutaneous infusion using a battery-operated syringe driver. Such a method delivers a dilute solution at a controlled dose and rate over 24 hours, maintaining a pain-free state. The oral starting dose is 0.5 mg/kg/24 hr in 4-hourly doses. A little persuasion may be needed for the subcutaneous route as a fine needle is used, and at some stage a well-meaning person may have promised 'no more injections'. While this method removes the need for regular injections the site of the needle puncture needs to be inspected frequently. There could be poor absorption after a while as there can be local crystallising of the drug, and the needle needs to be re-sited. In some instances it may be appropriate to add diazepam, promazine or chlorpromazine to help relieve anxiety or stress which enhances pain or vomiting. Should a central venous line be in situ, this route may also be considered for giving analgesia and other appropriate drugs.

Constipation

Constipation is a particular problem with opiates, which may be made worse by a poor dietary and fluid intake. Regular lactulose will help, but senna or suppositories may be needed.

Palliation

The site of the cancer may be such that it causes pressure pain, respiratory distress, etc. Palliative radiotherapy may be very appropriate in such cases if the tumour is radiosensitive. Similarly, steroids might help with bone pain. Since these methods were included in the treatment therapies, a careful explanation as to their new role must be given.

Vomiting

Vomiting is very distressing for the child and carers alike. It may be that anti-emetics which were effective during therapy cease to be so, or conversely that a previously non-effective agent now comes into its own. The most effective control may only be achieved by 'trial and error', each child being very different. It is essential that thirst, a sometimes distressing problem, is avoided, and nasogastric feeding or intravenous alimentation may be needed.

Bruising and Bleeding

It is not uncommon for platelet transfusion to be needed in order to prevent bleeding becoming a very real problem. Blood transfusion may be very pertinent and should not be denied during the terminal phase. Children look and feel better after transfusion, and although shortlived it is a valuable palliative therapy.

Infection

Infection in any form can be distressing to the child and most infections should be treated. The terminal state is no reason to think that a painful, distressing pneumonia or abscess should not be relieved and the child returned to a better quality of life. Similarly, due consideration must be given to anti-bacterial therapy, to ensure that it does not add diarrhoea to the child's other problems.

Sore Mouth

Encouraging a good diet and a high fluid intake is necessary to prevent a sore mouth. Oral hygiene and dental care need to be conscientiously attended to.

Fear

Fear in a child may show in different ways – not asking questions, asking everything numerous times, complaining of some non-existent problem, or saying 'I want my mummy' when she is there. Children cannot be made to talk about things they do not want to, but one can provide the opportunity – the right person (his choice) with time, and in the right environment using play. 'Am I going to die?' Does he want to know that he will or will not die? 'We all die sometime. What makes you ask, is something bothering you?' It can be a relief to be allowed to be scared when trying to be brave. One should not presume that one understands the thought behind the question, it could be entirely different from one's own thought, so it is wise to clarify the question. For example: (Child) 'I think I'm dying.' (Nurse) 'What makes you say that?' (Child) 'My mummy says that she's dying when she's got a tummy pain, and I've got a tummy pain.' Carers should not jump to conclusions. The most junior nurse is vulnerable to the unexpected question, as she seems readily available. She may have an advantage in saying 'I don't know, but I'll go and ask', but then she *must* return with an answer. It took courage to ask the question and so it should be respected and given a simple but honest response. Eye-to-eye contact is very important and noticeable if absent.

Such questions and the responses given should be disclosed to the parents, so that the handling of the child may be consistent. There is no point in one person denying death, if another has said that it is a real possibility. Individuals should not make promises that cannot be kept, like 'no more injections', as therapies change. Everyone should tell the same story. If a member of the caring team is anxious about something they have said, they must admit it to a colleague who can sort out the confusion.

Touch is a vital communicator, and even the older child might yearn for a cuddle. Praise for small achievements is encouraging. Honesty between parent and child that death is inevitable is very painful, but can relieve the distress of not knowing what is happening for the child. A calmness can result and more be gained from each other's company. The child then has the opportunity to ask what death is like, and whether it hurts. It could be that the child only wants to talk about death to one parent, the other being left to hold up the pretence as before. The family's coping system should be respected. A family is coping well when they are able to meet the demands of daily living despite the stressed circumstances.

CHILD'S UNDERSTANDING

A child's understanding of what is going on in terms of his own mortality will vary with age, stage of development and his previous experience (see Table 11.1). There is little appreciation before two years of age when the child faces the idea of death with simplicity and logic. A child who has lost a favourite grandparent or pet may possibly have an understanding that when you die you live on in another place where everyone goes and your then useless body is discarded. After about six years of age the child has a greater understanding of death, and by eight years the finality of death is understood. The young can have fanciful ideas about death, what it is like and what happens. In order to respond to the child's questions, the listener must enquire as to his opinion to guide the reply. An honest response to 'Where is . . . ?' (who has not been seen at the clinic) should be given. Sometimes the courage to be honest fails the parent – a child suspected that a fellow patient had died and had not been moved elsewhere as his mother had said. When he enquired as to the whereabouts of another child, he was told again that he had been moved. He said: 'Are you telling me the same lie you told me before?' Later his mother was able to respect his knowledge of the reality and they were able to talk about his own imminent death.

Many children know they are going to die, perhaps indicating this in their play or conversation in a matter-of-fact fashion which can be somewhat disarming. 'Do you want to hear a joke? I'm going home today with my drip.' This child died later that day. Some children know but do not want their parents to know. They have seen their parents suffer whenever their illness is mentioned, and not wishing to hurt them further, might say: 'Don't cry. Mum, I'll be all right, I'll be good.' At the same time the parent is trying to protect the child from knowing. How better can this point be made than in Anne Mary McPake's poignant verses which her parents have so graciously allowed to be included here (see p.166).

Spiritual Support

Respecting the views of the family, it may fall to the nurse to offer to contact a spiritual adviser of their choice, or one nominated by the hospital. A nurse must never impose her own views without permission from the parents. Not only does the spiritual advisor give religious support, but offers support from someone who has little to do with treatment.

DEATH

As the time passes parents may become very possessive of the time that is left with their child. Professionals, in their concern for the welfare of the parents, need to bear in mind that being there at the end is very important. However, it can be very difficult to judge the remaining hours.

Most expected deaths are calm and unhurried. The phase of dying slips, however briefly, into semi-consciousness, when communication seems impossible. Our first experience at birth is the sense of touch, and from then much is conveyed through it: the caress, cuddle and even the handshake. At no time is it more important to give as well as to receive than when someone is dying, as it shows that one is cared for.

Those who have seen death before develop a 'hunch' for when the child is about to die, but there is never absolute certainty as to when. The child may have been talking calmly, then seems to slip into sleep, respiration becoming increasingly shallow until the relaxation that follows is the moment of death. It is unfortunate that for some the breathing is laboured and hard-fought for, or there might be uncontrollable bleeding or persistent incontinence with accompanying distress. However, in most cases death is peaceful, with pain and symptoms well controlled.

Following the child's death there are practicalities that require attention, such as calling a doctor to certify that death has taken place. This does not mean that the parents need to be rushed away. They need time to say goodbye, time to realise that there are other family members to contact. Nurses must sensitively continue to support parents, perhaps offering to make an important telephone call for them. Do the parents want to participate in the last act of washing and dressing their child? What are their wishes regarding clothing and accompanying items such as a favourite toy? The question of post-mortem might well have been discussed earlier if the opportunity had presented itself, and the doctor may not be faced with the sensitive task of asking such a painful question at this time. However, if the answer is not known, such a request should be made before the parents leave the hospital.

It is well to remember that what is said and how one behaves are important to the parents, as they will remember this time for the rest of their lives. Saying, sincerely, 'I'm sorry' with a hand on the parent's shoulder, non-verbal expressions and the tone of voice saying the rest is all that may be required. Should the parents see how nurse feels? There is nothing wrong with a few tears being shed – the nurse's role is to support, to face practicalities and not to forget the other children and parents in the ward and to be in control.

There are some very unhelpful words that are sometimes said in an effort to console the bereaved: 'Never mind, it's for the best', 'You'll get over it', 'You can have another child/at least you have another child.'

Parents do not like the idea that their child will be on his own and efforts should be made for a nurse to stay with the child while he is in the ward. Leaving their child behind is very difficult. There is little need to rush parents. They should not leave the hospital on their own unless they express a wish to, or there is no alternative. The hospital doctor or nurse should telephone the GP, the health visitor or appropriate person, to inform them of the child's death and that the parents are on their way home.

The child can be visited in the hospital chapel. The parents may indicate who they want to see the child, for example, grandparents or other relatives. Sensitivity and flexibility will be required of staff in order for such visits to be as undistressing as possible. The nurse-in-charge needs to be sensitive to the feelings of others on duty, other parents and children. Attention could well be needed at some point for the expression of feelings and the answering of questions.

The death of a child in the ward affects everyone. In order that team members are not 'caught unawares' someone should ensure that everyone has been informed of what has happened before returning to the ward. Such preparation allows professionals to be more supportive of each other.

Eternal Life

Death is not the final parting
From the people we hold dear,
But a journey to another place
That holds no strain or fear.

It's the start of many meetings
With our loved ones gone before,
It's a way to lasting happiness
Through Paradise's door.

For the family that is left
There's a feeling of such pain,
The fear the one they loved
Will ne'er live to love again.

But someday God's voice will call you
To his garden up above,
To share with him 'Eternal Life',
And join your loss in love.

Anne Mary McPake, aged 14 years
(Written a few months before she died in 1987, with thanks to her parents)

References

Hall M, Hardin K and Conatser C (1982) The challenges of psychological care. In: *Nursing Care of the Child with Cancer*, Fotchman D and Foley G (eds.) Boston: Little, Brown.

Further Reading

Dominica Mother F (1987) Reflections of death in childhood. *British Medical Journal*, **294**: 108-110.

James J A, Harris D J, Mott M G and Oakhill A (1988) Paediatric oncology information pack for general practitioners. *British Medical Journal*, **296:** 97-98.

Kubler-Ross E (1983) *On Children and Death.* New York: Macmillan.

Muller D J, Harris P J and Wattley L (1986) *Nursing Children Psychology and Practice.* London: Harper and Row.

Regnard C F B and Davies A (1986) *Sympton Relief in Advanced Cancer.* Manchester: Haigh and Hochland Ltd.

Ward P and Oakhill A (1988) Terminal care. In: *The Supportive Care of the Child with Cancer*, Oakhill A. London: Wright.

12

Teamwork – Caring for the Child, the Family and the Staff

It is recognised that the successful management of a child with cancer and his family requires understanding and cooperation from a variety of health care professionals working together as a team. The aim of this chapter is to give a brief overview of the role of the various members who make up the multidisciplinary team. Each hospital or unit will have its own unique team and individuals may adopt a different or additional role to cover those areas where there is no appropriately qualified person. (There is no priority or significance to the order in which they appear.) The role of some members of the team will have been discussed in previous chapters.

The *Concise Oxford Dictionary* describes the word 'team' as 'two or more beasts of burden harnessed together'. It describes 'team work' as 'a combined effort or organised cooperation'. The first description is an example of a more traditional, old-fashioned team system. The team – the harnessed animals – need someone to direct them/drive them and has an object or load to be directed or moved. There is no indication that the team play an active part, or are involved in or agree in any way, in the decision-making of the actual goal. The second description – the combined effort of organised cooperation – is a much better explanation of teamwork and providing that the child and his family are encouraged and educated, they are more likely to be able to cooperate in the planning of realistic goals and assist in achieving them. The multidisciplinary team has evolved as a necessity following the improvement in the treatment of childhood cancer. The treatments, be they curative or palliative, make great demands both physically and psychologically on the child and psychologically and financially on the family. The child and his family require help from all members of the team if they are to be active members themselves.

The Appendix to this chapter identifies the variety of staff that may be involved as members of the multidisciplinary team.

It is unlikely that all hospital units will have access to all input from all of these departments, but they signify the potential area of need by the child and his family and other members of the team.

The Appendix also identifies other departments that may have a direct effect upon the child and his family while in hospital. Departments indirectly involved with care of the child require information about the decisions made by the team and about individual children if they are to participate and are required to cooperate with requests for individualised treatment regimes. We must not presume that others will view the child patient with the same compassion and empathy if their workload is heavy or a procedure will take twice the length of the time as normal, just because it is a child with cancer. If these personnel are involved in the problem-solving approach of undertaking a procedure without frightening or causing pain to the child or imposing too much on the individual or the department it should result in a greater understanding and a far more comfortable working relationship.

THE TEAM

The most important members of the team are the child and his family. It is important to remember that the child and his family must be involved with assessing problems and needs associated with the disease and subsequent treatment, the setting of realistic goals of care and the evaluation of the care planned. With children and adolescents it is unlikely that they will cooperate with the team if they have not had a say in the decision-making and do not understand what the realistic goals are, or if the goal posts are moved without their being informed. The child's primary nurse is also another key person and her role has been discussed in previous chapters. It is worth stressing again, however, that the primary nurse is seen as the patient's advocate and at the time of diagnosis may be the communicator and facilitator with different members of the team until the parents and child are ready to participate with them. The primary nurse can assess the appropriate time for individuals of the team to be introduced rather than them all introducing themselves within the first few days in hospital.

The physician, surgeon and radiotherapist, as members of the paediatric oncology team, are used to working together – the diagnostic and treatment modalities require this. Each has his own area of expertise but none can truly care for the whole child in isolation. Children must be referred to the paediatrician, but as in the case of a child with leukaemia, he will be required to meet the haematologist, paediatric oncologist and radio-therapist as diagnosis is confirmed and treatment progresses. All the specialists of the paediatric team are responsible for the overall clinical management of the patient. Effective commun-ication between colleagues and the child and his family is vital. Although it may be daunting at first to be faced with several specialists, the parents and child are usually quick to acknowl-edge the essential input by each one. Communication between paediatric oncology centres is also vital if clinical trials and research programmes undertaken in each centre are to be evaluated and improved treatment protocols are to be formu-lated. When available, parents and children find information booklets about the roles of the different specialists, their name, the day and time of their ward rounds and clinic day, helpful.

Anaesthetic Staff

The anaesthetic team have an important role to play. Their involvement in assessing the feasibility of gaining the child's trust and cooperation, with or without the aid of sedation or anaesthesia, is required at diagnosis and again as the child and his family build up relationships with members of the team and gain experience and knowledge about the investigations and treatments and what is expected of them.

Social Worker

The role of the social worker will vary from hospital to hospital, depending upon resources and workload. The social worker assists the team by identifying needs within the family – the needs may be emotional, social or financial. Many centres now have paediatric social workers, often funded by charities, for example, The Malcolm Sargent Cancer Fund for Children, who are employed solely for the paediatric oncology unit. Social workers' training includes counselling and communication skills, knowledge of group and family dynamics, interpersonal re-lationships and knowledge of the availability of resources for the whole family. Their training enables them to establish relationships quickly, sensitively and effectively. They assist the family by assessing their needs and problems and supporting all family members as they learn to deal and cope with situations they confront.

To some families there may be a social stigma attached to being introduced to the social worker. It is therefore important that they are introduced as another member of the team, at the time of diagnosis, so that relationships can be established.

Social workers are not confined or restricted to working with the family in hospital, they visit the patient and family at home and in some centres may visit the patient's school to prepare teachers and fellow pupils for the child's return. The social worker can help with practical advice on coping with the rest of the family, helping parents to be aware of the important needs of siblings and making suitable arrangements for their lives to be disrupted as little as possible. This may include direct contact with the siblings and talking to teachers and children of the school that the siblings attend. Each family will have its own relationship with the social worker and their needs will vary as they go through the stages of investigation, diagnosis and treatment of their child's disease.

Social workers may organise or be involved in group work as support for parents, the children and the staff. Group activities may be targeted for specific reasons, for example, the family of a newly diagnosed child with cancer, or families facing the cessation of treatment, or following bereavement.

The social worker is identified as being a non-threatening member of the team, neither medical or nursing and not associated with painful or unpleasant procedures. This therefore, enables the social worker to be accepted as a supporter for the whole family.

The Chaplain/Religious Leaders

The religious beliefs and spiritual needs of each child and family will vary and change. The chaplain needs to be seen as a member of the team who is on the ward regularly as a friend providing support, not just as a member or representative of the Church. Families with religious beliefs may want to use the chaplain individually or as a link person with their own local priest or minister. It is important that the different cultural and religious beliefs that ethnic minorities and overseas families may have are acknowledged and facilities are available to meet them. The chaplain may again be the mediator for this. The chaplain may also be involved in group support for parents and/or staff.

Psychologist/Psychiatrist

Many people perceive a stigma attached to receiving help or support from a psychologist or psychiatrist. For many families the support and help from the nurses, social workers and doctors is sufficient, others, however, may benefit from working with a psychologist or psychiatrist. Again, if these professionals are accepted as a member of the team and introduced to children and their families following the diagnosis of cancer, families will be helped to overcome their often negative thoughts, e.g. that the reason the psychologist is seeing them is because they are having problems, rather than having positive thoughts, e.g. this is someone else who can help me sort out my feelings of anger, despair, etc.

As well as helping the child and his family come to terms with the diagnosis of cancer, the psychologist/psychiatrist may also help the patient develop coping strategies to come to terms with the treatment and the limitations that this may pose, e.g. coping with time away from home, school and friends, repeated unpleasant and/or painful procedures while in hospital.

Siblings may also require help from the psychologist/ psychiatrist to cope with the emotional and family dynamic changes once the cancer is diagnosed and treatment begins. Again, this should not be seen in isolation but as part of helping the whole family survive emotionally throughout the treatment phase and beyond.

Staff may want to use these members of the team for support and help although again, even professionals may have problems relating to the psychologist and/or psychiatrist.

Physiotherapist

The physiotherapist's role in preventative medicine is as important as that of therapeutic treatments. Being based on the wards he can get to know the children and establish relationships with them. If the child should require physiotherapy he is then not faced with meeting yet another person who attempts to undertake uncomfortable procedures when he least feels like it. For children who face intensive treatment that renders them weak and unable to get out of bed for days or weeks, e.g. during bone marrow transplantation, routine deep breathing exercises and muscle exercises can be made into games and can be practised before the child becomes unwell following treatment. Having played with the child the physiotherapist is more likely to gain the child's cooperation. Visits to the gym for physiotherapy or just play acts as diversional therapy for the child and may also give the parents an opportunity to have a break.

Dietitian/Nutritionalist

From the moment children are born, mothers are concerned about their nourishment. Parents are often heard to say, 'He hasn't eaten anything today' or 'I can't get him to eat anything'. The dietitian or nutritionalist can help by working with the child and his parents, finding out the type of foods the child normally eats, what he fancies when he is ill and what he dislikes especially when receiving treatment. By knowing the treatment that the child is to receive and the possible side-effects, the dietitian can work with the family in maintaining the patient's weight and appetite despite the disease and its treatment. Providing facilities on the ward for parents to prepare and cook food for their children is of great benefit. This enables children to have what they like when they want it and if it is mum or dad's cooking it is also often much more acceptable. The dietitian can work with the parents in making the treat or snack more nutritious or, in the case of children on steroids with weight problems, help in reducing the calorific intake without making the food unappetising.

Again, by being part of the team and knowing the long-term plan for the patient, the dietitian can help the parents to prepare and cope with the dietary problems that the disease and its treatment may cause.

Play Therapist

Children view the play therapist as the most important member of the ward team. Traditionally, the play therapist was someone who kept young children occupied, gave them things do to pass away the time and stopped them thinking about their treatment, operation or the fact their parents were not on the ward.

Today their role has developed much more. The therapy part is as important as the play. Appropriately qualified play therapists can help prepare children of all age groups for their treatments, haematological investigations, bone marrow aspiration, anaesthesia, central venous line care, radiotherapy, etc. By playing with toys, dolls and using safe equipment such as blood pressure cuffs, syringes and bandages, the children have the opportunity to act out their fears, anxieties, aggression and other feelings.

The play therapist may also be of help to siblings when they visit, again by providing an accepting environment for them to act out how they are feeling. The play therapist needs to be an active member of the team if she is to assist in the preparation of the children effectively for their treatments. She must feel comfortable in her role and free to liaise with medical and nursing colleagues about the problems children may exhibit through play. The play therapist may also work alongside the physiotherapist or the dietitian in providing play activities for the preventative or therapeutic elements of their treatment, for example, organising cooking activities for the children having liaised with the dietitian as to the nutritional requirements for items to be cooked and hopefully eaten.

The play therapist's skills are also required in the outpatient department to help prevent anxieties and fears building up while children are waiting for haematological investigations and other planned diagnostic or treatment procedures.

School Teacher

Facilities should be available for children to continue their education when in hospital, especially for those who are going to be in hospital for some time. Again, a school teacher needs to be aware of the various treatments that the children are having and the limitations such treatments may put on their school work while they are in hospital. Having direct contact with the team she will be able to organise her day and the child's day by knowing the most convenient time of the day to plan her session with the individual child. Links with the child's own school and school teacher should also be encouraged.

The Extended Team

Other important members of the team include the ward clerk or receptionist, domestic staff, porters, research personnel and secretarial staff. They all have a significant role to play and if they are to undertake that role efficiently and effectively they need to feel part of the team and understand the unit's philosophy and aims.

Domestic staff require an understanding of the 'special' procedures on the ward, for example, reverse barrier nursing and radioactive iodine treatment, which affect how and when they can undertake their work. Knowing the rationale behind the ward policies, parents cooking for the child and themselves and being kept up to date with the different events on the ward can aid in planning the day more efficiently and working as a member of the team.

The ward clerk is often the first person the child and parents come into contact with on the ward and by telephone. She is often the one who liaises with other departments searching for results, requesting appointments, etc. To help her assist the child and his family and to explain the ward philosophy to other departments, she needs to be involved with the team, and information concerning decisions about the children, the ward, etc. should be shared with her. This also applies to the research and secretarial staff. They all get to know the children and their families for different reasons and in different capacities. If they are to function efficiently and support the ward and all its beliefs, then they need to be involved, included and valued.

Indirect Members of the Team

These are members of the team who also have a vital role to play but are often not involved in decision-making about planned treatments. They are the people involved in other departments. Communication and negotiation is vital if their cooperation and support is to continue. Routine investigations may take longer if time has to be allowed to let a child relax and cooperate. Procedures that may normally take 20 minutes may take twice the length of time if the patient requires an anaesthetic and other painful or invasive investigations are then performed under the same anaesthetic.

If the ward philosophy and the individual needs of the child are shared with the staff in the various departments, agreement is more likely to be reached in planning individualised approaches to care that are acceptable and workable to all.

CARING FOR THE TEAM

So far we have examined the needs of the children and their families, but what about the needs of the carers? Working with children with cancer and their families is stressful. Health care professionals working in this field need to be able to develop effective coping mechanisms and avoid or prevent stressful situations occurring. How can this be achieved? Staff support can be considered in two ways:

- *Organisational support*, adequate staffing levels, correct skill mix, up-to-date equipment in working order, and an environment that is conducive with a clearly stated ward philosophy.
- *Interpersonal support*, support from one colleague to another.

The National Health Service finds it difficult in the present financial climate to maintain its resources. It is therefore important that good interpersonal support is achieved to prevent emotional detachment and burnout.

Caring for children with cancer has brought additional stresses in the last decade. The alteration in treatment programmes and the introduction of family-centred care and primary nursing encourages nurses to become more involved with the whole family and to accept more responsibility.

Are there signs to recognise that staff are no longer coping? Chernis (1980) and Marshall (1980) indicate that staff who do not have interpersonal support develop coping strategies which may affect their work performance, directly or indirectly. These coping strategies may be in the form of emotional detachment, ineffectual rationalisation, or an inappropriate sense of humour, altered goals and an altered sense of responsibility. Chernis (1980) describes the above as burnout, Marshall (1980) as emotional detachment. Interpersonal relationships have to be effective if one is going to be able to recognise any of the above signs. Burnout or emotional detachment can happen to the most experienced staff as well as newly qualified staff and is probably due to the lack of emotional support from both peers and the hierarchy.

What constitutes good support? What are the ingredients? Pines and Aronson (1981) describe it as alternative listening, communicating, appreciation of others' abilities, encouragement of critical thinking and emotional support. Chernis (1980) describes it as a feedback on performance – appraisal, opportunity to update and gain new information – study days/nursing conferences, emotional support and opportunity for the venting of feelings. One area common to both the above findings is emotional support.

Support starts at peer level on the ward on a day-to-day basis. Relationships between staff need to be well established. The environment needs to be conducive for individuals to be able to say thank you, please and help, not just for physical things but emotional needs as well. To be able to do this nurses need to be taught, during their training, the importance of empathy, respect and honesty in relationships with each other, so that when they reach staff nurse, sister/charge nurse level they have the skills to cope. They do not have to learn the hard way, developing their own coping mechanisms while helping others to develop theirs.

Making people feel involved and appreciated is also essential in providing emotional support. Involving all personnel in decision-making is associated with a higher morale. Primary nursing is an example of this, the responsibility of assessing, planning, implementing, and evaluating the care of the child with him and his family has helped to increase nurses' feeling of job satisfaction.

Support sessions can be formal or informal. They can be one-to-one or in a group. Individuals within the team will have different ways of giving and receiving support. Some may find it difficult to work in groups, others may find group support more beneficial. Members of a team with specific training in group dynamics and counselling skills may be the appropriate facilitator of support groups, e.g. the social worker, the chaplain or the psychologist/psychiatrist.

When planning a group ground-rules or parameters may have to be set; these would include:

- Are all staff required to attend?
- Do different levels of trained staff require different groups? For example, one for the students and one for the trained staff?
- When will they be held, on- or off-duty?
- Where will they be held – on or off the ward?
- How long will the meeting last?
- How often?

The needs of the group will also have to be identified in order:

- To help clarify how the participants will use the group
- To help the group leader focus on the appropriate needs of the group
- To identify boundaries, to eliminate expectations and needs which cannot be met
- To help participants see that the success of the group is shared responsibility between themselves and the leader

- To establish a safe and confidential atmosphere
- To decide upon the format: group topic, calling for individual expression, case presentation, etc.
- To decide how many meetings and how to evaluate them

If the groups are to be formal the qualities of the leader or the facilitator must be considered. Appropriate qualities would include:

- The ability to communicate empathy
- To be able to communicate respect
- To be congruent
- To be concrete
- To be confident
- Reflect, clarify and draw relevant points together
- Be supportive
- Be relaxed
- Have a sense of humour
- Have the ability to help every member to contribute – using and being aware of verbal and *non* verbal communication.

Not all members of the staff may be comfortable using a group session but they may use the facilitators of such a group as a one-to-one support.

Problems within the team may occur and cause additional stress. These problems may be due to role conflict, different ethical beliefs, different philosophical beliefs and different coping strategies. Conflicts such as these need to be identified, discussed and individual roles clarified.

Members of the team need reassurance that stress is not a disease, it is a natural response to threats to our physical and psychological well-being. Responses of anger, disgust, grief and fear are normal, it is only when they become prolonged that the warning bells should sound. It is well documented that play is an important ingredient for child development. It is also an important ingredient for staff support. Kuykendall (1988) says, 'let us not be afraid to play'. His statement is related to children. It should be extended to staff: celebrations for the child coming out of isolation, or discharge after a long admission period, birthdays for staff, patients and relatives, engagements or just to cheer everybody up. Staff need to be able to laugh together, as well as cry together.

Other methods of helping to relieve and reduce stress may include relaxation, meditation and exercise. Again, this can be a group or ward activity.

Storlie (1979) comments that nurses working with patients with cancer have been identified as a group with a high risk of experiencing burnout. Shubin (1978) cautions nurses to be alert for early signs of burnout so that appropriate interventions can be made.

Despite the problems of stress, working with children with cancer and their families is very rewarding. A cohesive team approach offers the best chance of providing a stable and trusting environment to make the patient and family feel cared for and supported. Providing there is trust and respect from one's colleagues, it should also form a means of support for each member of the team.

APPENDIX
THE TEAM, CHILD AND HIS FAMILY

Paediatrician
Primary nurse/associate
Oncologist
Haematologist
Surgeon
Radiotherapist
Anaesthetist
Psychologist/psychiatrist
School teacher
Community paediatric nurse

School nurse
General practitioner
Social worker
Community liaison nurse
Sister/charge nurse
Chaplain
Physiotherapist
Nutritionalist
Dietitian
Play therapist
Health visitor

EXTENDED TEAM

Domestic staff
Ward clerk
Secretarial staff
Research personnel

INDIRECT MEMBERS OF THE TEAM

Radiographers
Pharmacists
Ambulance staff

Mould room technicians
Catering staff
Portering staff

References

Chernis G (1980) *Professional Burnout in Human Service Organisations.* New York: Praeger.

Kuykendall J (1988) Play therapy. In: *The Supportive Care of the Child with Cancer*, Oakhill A (ed.), chapter 11. Guildford: Butterworth.

Marshall J (1980) Stress amongst nurses. In: *White Collar and Professional Stress*, Cooper C L and Marshall J (eds.). New York: John Wiley.

Pines A and Aronson E (1981) *Burnout: Team Tedium to Personal Growth.* New York: Free Press.

Shubin S (1978) Burnout: the professional hazard you face. *Nursing,* **8:** 722.

Storlie F J (1979) Burnout: the elaboration of a concept. *American Journal of Nursing.* **79:** 2108-2111.

Further Reading

Bond M (1982) Do you care about your colleagues? Stress 4. *Nursing Mirror,* **155**(16): 42-44.

Fotchman D and Foley G (1982) *Nursing Care of the Child with Cancer.* Boston: Little, Brown.

Oakhill A (1988) *Supportive Care of the Child with Cancer.* London: Wright.

Index

Index prepared by Sara Firman.